Praise for *Heal Your Pain Now*

"This book will help people who suffer from chronic pain from co[nditions] such as fibromyalgia, autoimmune disease, musculo[skeletal injury], or any persistent pain state. Dr. Joe Tatta has written a blueprint to [heal] pain using integrated, functional medicine principles. I recomme[nd this] book and the Healing Pain Program."

> —Mark Hyman, MD, #1 *New York Times* bestselling author
> of *The Blood Sugar Solution 10-Day Detox Diet*

"We've been approaching pain all wrong. The solution doesn't come in a bottle; it comes by taking control of your health. Dr. Tatta provides a simple, easy-to-implement strategy that helps you break free from pain and live the life you deserve."

> —JJ Virgin, *New York Times* bestselling author of *JJ Virgin's Sugar
> Impact Diet* and *The Virgin Diet*

"Dr. Tatta is a rare breed of physical therapist, nutritionist, and functional medicine practitioner. This book provides easy, effective strategies and natural strategies for those who want to heal their pain."

> —Dr. Alan Christianson, *New York Times* bestselling author
> of *The Adrenal Reset Diet*

"If persistent pain is holding you hostage, let Dr. Joe Tatta show you how to break free! Through his amazing Healing Pain Program, he's helped thousands of people reclaim their lives—and now it's your turn."

> —Dr. Kellyann Petrucci, *New York Times* bestselling author of
> *Dr. Kellyann's Bone Broth Diet* and host of the Public Television
> Special "21 Days to a Slimmer, Younger You!"

"At last—a must read book for those who struggle with pain. *Heal Your Pain Now* mindfully brings readers through an amazing healing journey. Dr. Tatta shows you how emotions and thoughts are right at the core of your pain experience. He outlines practical and concrete ways you can use the power of your mind to reverse pain. This book is also a much needed resource for health care professional who want to help patients successfully cope and thrive!"

> —Dr. Susan Albers, *New York Times* bestselling author of *Eat.Q.*

"Dr. Tatta has compiled a trove of the latest information about pain. More importantly, he has distilled this information into an evidence-based program that has helped many people overcome their pain. I highly recommend this book."

> —Howard Schubiner, MD, author of *Unlearn Your Pain* and *Unlearn
> Your Anxiety and Depression*; Providence Hospital, Southfield, MI

"*Heal Your Pain Now* addresses the current global pain epidemic with Dr. Tatta's integrated approach—starting with the gut microbiome and ending with the latest advances in how your brain processes pain. The book will uncover the root cause(s) of your pain and help you develop a plan for healing naturally. I have experienced the power of Dr. Tatta's work myself. If you have chronic or persistent pain that no one has been able to resolve, this book is a must read! It is the template to your pain healing journey."

> —Dr. Vincent Pedre, MD, Certified Functional Medicine Practitioner and author of *Happy Gut: The Cleansing Program To Help You Lose Weight, Gain Energy, and Eliminate Pain*

"Dr. Tatta provides important perspectives in *Heal Your Pain Now* on the role of weight loss, nutrition for pain relief, the role of the brain in pain, pain 'catastrophizing,' breathing exercises for stress, strength and posture activities, and much more. I applaud his efforts and his passion for his patients and his readers' overall health and well-being."

> —David Schechter, MD, Sports Medicine/Chronic Pain Specialist, Beverly Hills, CA, and author of *Think Away Your Pain* and *The MindBody Workbook*

"Dr. Tatta is one of the few who understand and articulate the full complexity of chronic pain syndromes, including the concept that while much of chronic pain is driven by factors such as inflammation and tissue trauma, some is not! His explanation of brain-derived and emotional pain and central sensitization are spot-on! His support program, full of comprehensive integrative tools needed to heal from persistent pain are delivered in an easy to follow program. This book is a must read for anyone suffering with chronic pain."

> —Dr. David Brady, ND, author of *The Fibro Fix*

"Dr. Tatta has turned his immense energy, passion, and professional training into a remarkably user-friendly and practical book designed to help people who struggle with chronic pain. In this day of hyper-specialization and fragmented messages within health care, he has filled an important gap by combining his clinical experience as a physical therapist with training in nutrition and new information from the pain sciences. He presents a holistic approach that goes well beyond typical clinical care, helping those who suffer to get their lives back on track and move toward health."

> —Dr. Phil McClure, PT, PhD, Professor and Chair, Arcadia University, Department of Physical Therapy

HEAL YOUR PAIN NOW

HEAL
Your Pain
NOW

The Revolutionary Program to Reset
Your Brain and Body for a Pain-Free Life

Dr. Joe Tatta, DPT, CNS

Da Capo
LIFE
LONG

Copyright © 2017 by Joe Tatta

Photographs by Bill Westmoreland

Designed by Trish Wilkinson
Set in 11.25-point Adobe Caslon Pro by Perseus Books

Cataloging-in-Publication data for this book is available from the Library of Congress.

First Da Capo Press edition 2017
ISBN: 978-0-7382-1922-6 (paperback)
ISBN: 978-0-7382-1923-3 (e-book)

Published by Da Capo Press, an imprint of Perseus Books, LLC, a subsidiary of Hachette Book Group, Inc.

www.dacapopress.com

Da Capo Press books are available at special discounts for bulk purchases in the U.S. by corporations, institutions, and other organizations. For more information, please contact the Special Markets Department at Perseus Books, 2300 Chestnut Street, Suite 200, Philadelphia, PA 19103, or call (800) 810-4145, ext. 5000, or e-mail special .markets@perseusbooks.com.

10 9 8 7 6 5 4 3 2 1

*For Jeorge who has taught me that love
is the most powerful force in healing*

CONTENTS

FOREWORD

Who hasn't experienced pain at some point in their life? As a medical doctor who practices functional medicine for mostly women, I routinely see how pain impacts people on every level, from mildly uncomfortable to miserable.

Conventional medicine's approach to pain is outdated. Over the past decade, cutting-edge science has redefined pain and how to treat it effectively. Simply put, pain serves as an alarm to get your attention. That alarm can be empowering, because it shifts the power to heal into your own hands.

Over decades of practicing functional medicine for women, I've learned women report more pain than men do. Stress plays a role, particularly in pain related to the gastrointestinal system and fibromyalgia, and women experience more stress compared with men.* An estimated 25 percent of Americans experience chronic pain, and a disproportionate number of them are women.

One review published in the *Journal of Pain* found women faced a substantially greater risk of developing persistent pain syndromes. Researchers here found women are twice as likely to have multiple sclerosis, two to three times more likely to develop rheumatoid arthritis,

---

*M. Million et al., "Stress, Sex, and the Enteric Nervous System." *Neurogastroenterology & Motility* 28, no. 9 (2016): 1283–89; S. Fischer et al., "Stress Exacerbates Pain in the Everyday Lives of Women with Fibromyalgia Syndrome—The Role of Cortisol and Alpha-Amylase." *Psychoneuroendocrinology* 63 (2016): 68–77; "Stress in America," American Psychological Association, accessed August 31, 2016, http://www.apa.org/news/press/releases/stress/.

and four times more likely to have chronic fatigue syndrome than are men. Autoimmune diseases, which include debilitating pain, strike women three to four times more frequently than they do men.*

Likewise, the Institute of Medicine published a report on the public health impact of chronic pain, which reported that women suffered more from pain. Equally disturbing, doctors were more likely to dismiss those pain reports.†

When they *are* diagnosed, women are less likely to receive aggressive treatment. Many doctors instead characterize their pain as "psychogenic" and, therefore, "not real." Let me be completely clear: Your pain is real. It doesn't just exist "in your head." You are not crazy or delusional.

When I work with patients, I diagnose and treat on complete trust in the person reporting those symptoms. Measuring pain is difficult because it's subjective and depends on self-reporting. To assume that my female patients exaggerate that pain would be deeply offensive and, honestly, misogynistic.

From a biochemical-individuality premise where everyone is unique, my friend Dr. Joe Tatta wrote *Heal Your Pain Now* to initiate your healing journey. Within these pages, you'll discover how to approach pain as an emotional and sensory experience, and equally important, to implement the right healing strategies that alleviate pain.

This groundbreaking book rests on a fundamental but overlooked principle: Your brain, *not* your body, creates pain. That might sound simple, but practitioners often disregard that idea.

Beginning with an evaluation about why past treatments probably failed you (trust me: It's *not* your fault), Dr. Tatta implements the latest pain-science–based research to show how incorporating such

---

*"Autoimmune Disease in Women," American Autoimmune Related Diseases Association, https://www.aarda.org/autoimmune-information/autoimmune -disease-in-women/.

†Institute of Medicine: Committee on Advancing Pain Research, Care, and Education, *Relieving Pain in America: A Blueprint for Transforming Prevention, Care, Education, and Research.* (Washington, DC: National Academies Press, 2011).

things as nutrition, gut health, weight loss, exercise, and education about the pain experience can become part of a customized protocol to heal your pain.

I love how practical and easy to implement these tools (the same ones I use in my own practice) are to lose weight, create your healthiest self, and eliminate the pain that holds your happiness and life hostage. Dr. Tatta even mentions my favorite form of movement—yoga—that research shows can decrease back pain,* neck pain,† and even autoimmune disease.‡

Ultimately, *Heal Your Pain Now* provides a well-researched, powerful guide to rewire your brain and alleviate pain immediately. Whether you only recently began suffering or struggled miserably with pain for years, consider this book your go-to source to find relief and create the vibrant, healthy life you were meant to live.

Sara Gottfried, MD
Berkeley, CA
Author of the *New York Times*
bestselling books *The Hormone Cure*
and *The Hormone Reset Diet*

---

*H. E. Tilbrook et al., "Yoga for Chronic Low Back Pain: A Randomized Trial," *Annals of Internal Medicine* 155, no. 9 (2011): 569–78.

†A. Michalsen et al., "Yoga for Chronic Neck Pain: A Pilot Randomized Controlled Clinical Trial." *Journal of Pain* 13, no. 11 (2012): 1122–30.

‡P. Sengupta, "Health Impacts of Yoga and Pranayama: A State-of-the-Art Review." *International Journal of Preventive Medicine* 3, no. 7 (2012).

INTRODUCTION

Mark was a forty-five-year-old professional who suffered with persistent pain in his neck and arm from an accident on his motorcycle more than ten years ago. He had broken a few bones and had been badly bruised, but his bumps and breaks were well healed by now—yet Mark was still in pain. We met at a party held by a mutual friend in a swanky Park Avenue apartment. The views of the city were breathtaking, the food and wine wonderful. The attendees ranged from a mix of New York's ultrasuccessful professionals to the starving artist and all those in between. But the conversations at this party, as at many I had attended before, had a theme. For me parties often turn into occasions for collecting others' stories of pain. We each have our own unique story of pain.

Once people hear I am a doctor of physical therapy and help free people from a life of pain, three questions typically follow. First, *how do I get rid of this persistent pain?* It might be joint pain, an old injury, or a disease. It is often disrupting to their work, personal life, and enjoyment. Second, *how do I get in shape or lose weight?* This is not surprising since so many of us struggle with extra weight, and the obesity epidemic not only disables our body but also cripples the health of our economy and medical system. Third, there is always someone who throws down the gauntlet in frustration or desperation and says, *but I have tried everything and nothing has worked; why do I still have this pain?* Mark was no different.

Mark was your average guy with a full-time job, family, and friends. He loved his job as a mediator and was passionate about teaching individuals and corporations the skills necessary to solve problems in a peaceful, amicable way. Mediators are trained and experienced in dispute resolution. I asked Mark how he successfully brought people to a peaceful conclusion around difficult issues, such as a divorce or a heated workplace dispute involving employees and employers. He simply shrugged his shoulders and said there was only one way to solve a dispute: Provide both parties with as much information as possible and then guide and facilitate them through the process until they reach a resolution. Mediation revolves around *your* decisions, not the mediator's. The mediator provides various solutions to help you navigate the process as you select which path you want to take, but ultimately *you* make the decisions.

I then asked Mark what he currently did for his pain, and he said, "Well, my doctor gave me some pills to take. I don't like to take them too often because they don't make me feel very good, but I need them. Sometimes I feel like I'm getting addicted to them and stop taking them, but I eventually wind up going back. The doctors say surgery can't help me as the fractures healed well. I try to stay active because I know it's good for me, but I just can't seem to work out the way I used to! It's like I need to start all over again from square one some weeks. And I notice I am putting on weight. I should start running! That will take the weight off, right?"

Mark's wasn't the only story I encountered that night. There was someone with arthritis in her knee who kept overdoing it, a former Olympic gymnast wearing a back brace, a sales rep with crippling carpal tunnel syndrome, and someone recently diagnosed with lupus. By the way, no one at the party was over the age of fifty.

"So, how do you help people in pain?" Mark asked.

"Well, I like to provide them with as much information as possible and then guide them through the process until they feel happy with their outcome," I replied.

Health and wellness have been constant themes in my life. When I was three years old, I started participating in gymnastics, and the healthy habits I learned at that young age were imprinted for a lifetime.

Excelling in a sport that requires physical skill and mental determination taught me a lot, triggered my interest, and sparked my lifelong passion to help others achieve optimal health.

I was also fortunate to be raised and inspired by a great mom who was also a nurse. Growing up, I was intrigued by the medical texts and journals lying around the house. The seeds for health care were planted in me at a young age. However, my mom influenced me in more ways than one to pursue a path of helping people in pain. Just when I was old enough to realize how strong my mother was, I watched her struggle with illness. She worked at a hospital on the adolescent cancer floor. Most of her patients were between the ages of five and fifteen and were terminally ill with cancer. She worked the night shift from two to eight a.m., taking care of children in need, only to come home and take care of her own children, husband, and home—and she was juggling it all! However, the stress of being a caregiver to many can take its toll. Studies have shown us that caregivers have increased markers of stress hormones and inflammatory proteins circulating throughout their blood, and that can impact almost every system in the body.

One day Mom arrived home from work, just as I was heading out to school. She looked spent and her eyes were filled with tears. In her arms she held a picture sketched of a little boy on a go-cart, drawn by one of her favorite patients. She had borne the stress of working as a nurse on the night shift and sleeping at odd hours, and like many caregivers, her health suffered. She had digestive issues, fatigue, bounced between anxiety and depression, and was in pain—both physically and emotionally. Like most who struggle with chronic pain, she was in the prime of her life with responsibilities of house, work, and family. She worried not only about her health but also about those around her and saw her life slipping away. With the help of a friend, she chartered a new path back to health and transformed herself, using principles similar to those in this book. She rebounded, reeducated, and reengaged with life and went on to become the vice president of nursing for one of the largest home-care agencies in New York. And if you met her today, you would see a vibrant, strong, and beautiful woman, enjoying her retirement. However, witnessing my mom's experience left a mark and an undying curiosity in me as to what is the best way to help people in pain. The one advantage she had was education. She overcame her pain, and you can, too, with the information you will discover in this book.

My career as a doctor of physical therapy has exposed me to a variety of patients. My first job was in adult rehabilitation, where I helped people recover from strokes, joint replacements, neurologic diseases, and amputations. This was a rewarding experience, although I knew a hospital was not the right fit for me. I saw firsthand the complexities of our medical system and realized the majority of people needed support before they reached the rehabilitation stage. After working for a few years with athletes and backstage with Broadway dancers, I found myself working for one of the largest outpatient physical therapy practices in New York City. Here I not only treated people with pain but also managed the training process for new doctors of physical therapy hired, as well as doctoral interns from more than forty schools. This program encompasses my twenty-plus years of experience and training in physical therapy, nutrition, and functional medicine as well as the years of lessons learned from the thousands of patients I have healed and clinicians with whom I have trained and collaborated.

The Current State of Pain

If you struggle with persistent pain, you understand how it can impact your life. We live in a world full of pain—and many of the high-tech procedures and pills used fail those in pain. Women are more likely to suffer with a chronic pain condition than are men. Pain is the most common reason for a visit to a doctor of physical therapy, and pain in its myriad of forms consistently ranks as the #1 or #2 reason for visiting a primary care physician. The numbers on pain are staggering:

- Chronic pain affects more than 100 million Americans—that is more than diabetes, heart disease, and cancer combined!

- 90 percent of Americans will have back pain at least once in their life and 30 percent will go on to have chronic back pain.
- An estimated 52.5 million US adults (about 1 in 5) report having doctor-diagnosed arthritis. As the US population ages, the number of adults with arthritis is expected to increase sharply to 67 million by 2030.
- 50 million Americans have an autoimmune disorder, which causes pain. There are more than 80 autoimmune diseases for which pain is a major symptom.
- 30 million have diabetes.
- 30 million live with irritable bowel disease.
- 20 million Americans live with mood disorders.
- About 5 million people are affected by fibromyalgia, a chronic pain condition.
- 1 million deal with chronic fatigue syndrome.

Pain is everywhere and *your pain is real.* Quite often it's overwhelming, intimidating, and, at times, downright terrifying. We take our health for granted, until a physical limitation inhibits our regular, everyday movement. Then suddenly we are so completely aware of our pain and immobility that it becomes all-consuming. Perhaps you suffer from serious back pain and can no longer easily bend down to pick up an item you've dropped on the floor, so you stop trying altogether and you begin to lose even more flexibility. Or maybe you have a knee injury that causes you to limp when you walk, and you unconsciously stop bending your knee normally out of fear that it will ache. Or possibly you have one of the more than eighty autoimmune disorders that can affect multiple joints and multiple organ systems at once. If you are experiencing pain like this, it can be debilitating, and you may have quit exercising entirely, which has likely just made you feel worse and even more helpless.

The Pain/Weight-Gain Connection

Many of those people suffering with pain are also struggling with weight issues. Being overweight is a risk factor for a host of diseases—all which have the awful effect of pain. Arthritis, autoimmune diseases, fibromyalgia, diabetes, heart disease, and neurological and musculoskeletal diseases all contribute to the persistent pain syndromes and are higher in those who are overweight or obese. More than two thirds of Americans (245 million people) are overweight or obese. This nation is overweight and in pain, and it is physically, economically, and emotionally crippling us. The statistics are alarming and have a deep and lasting impact on our families, community, economy, and society:

- More than 2 in 3 adults are overweight; more than 1 in 3 adults are obese.
- More than 1 in 20 adults are considered to have *extreme* obesity.
- About 69 percent or 215 million Americans are overweight, with more than 78 million adult Americans considered obese.
- Chronic pain type syndromes are the most common cause of long-term disability—and obesity rates for adults with disabilities are 58 percent higher than for adults without disabilities.

Pain and weight gain are intimately connected: Persistent pain leads you to become more sedentary, avoiding the discomfort you now associate with moving your body. The longer you are immobile, the more weight you will gain. Fat begins to accumulate around your belly in toxic layers, sabotaging your efforts to be healthy. The steady addition of 10, 20, 30—even 100-plus—pounds of extra weight makes it harder to move, so you remain inactive, resignedly watching the scale creep higher.

Persistent pain is a modern plague holding you captive. This often leads to unresolved feelings around the experience of pain and toward those involved. You may feel there is nothing you can do, you hold grievances, and believe only a miracle can save you. Your pain is very real, and you are not imagining it.

Nutrition, Movement, and the Brain:
A Three-Step Functional Medicine Approach

As a doctor of physical therapy, I began my career with an intense focus on the structure and function of the human form. The health of our joints, strength and flexibility, and teaching healthy movement were the primary modalities I used. Movement is necessary to live a healthy, pain-free life and to manage weight. However, certain patients would fail, struggle, or plateau. I noticed the world around me changing . . . or should I say getting bigger and more painful. I saw where the real need existed—those struggling with persistent pain. I also saw that movement alone could not cure the problem.

Surplus weight and obesity were strong contributing factors to my patients' struggles with pain, and I began implementing proper nutrition in a more integrative approach to patient care. Combining healthy movement with nutritional strategies is not new and has been shown to help not only patients with persistent pain but also many chronic diseases. But even with the best nutrition and exercise advice, pain can persist. As I worked with patients, it became apparent to me that something was missing: the integration of how our brain, thoughts, and emotions influenced our pain. Mastery of one's mind-set was needed with many clients. They lived with attack thoughts that hindered their full potential for recovery. Later, my study of functional medicine further solidified my integration of movement, nutrition, and the mind into a treatment paradigm. This is not an equal one-third movement, one-third nutrition, one-third cognitive-training program. This is a framework you can follow as a guide, and you may require more emphasis in one area than another.

You Are Your Best Advocate

We have a large body of evidence-based medicine and research to support the foundation of this program. Almost 90 percent of the chronic conditions people struggle with that are treated by clinicians can be overcome by simple and inexpensive means. Behavior changes associated with diet, exercise, lifestyle, and mind-set have revealed dramatic and lasting effects. Health promotion—proactive healthy habits and preventive care—will be the way we heal in the future, as it occurs *before* disease takes hold. The most rapid way to transform your health and resolve your pain begins with providing you with the tools to succeed. In the old world you relied on the man in the white coat to help you "fix" the problem. In the new world *your* ability to collect, synthesize, and apply the necessary information related to your pain will be the fastest way to healing. This may require some energy, but it will save you time, effort, money, and pain (literally and figuratively).

When I tell patients my job is merely that of a *teacher and coach*, I often receive blank stares or raised eyebrows. One patient replied, "Well, you're a *doctor*—isn't there some way you can fix me?" Our society really has no formal system for teaching us about how to live a healthy life. Sure, schools have some basic health education classes but not nearly the amount needed to shift the trend of chronic disease. Most of us know more about how our cell phones work than the body we live in. But the more actively involved you become in your own treatment program with regard to what you choose to put into your body, how you move your body, and your thought patterns during recovery, the more you will achieve positive results. This book creates a path for you to begin the journey toward healing your pain. For some your journey will be fast and your pain will be healed now; for others you will have to spend some time cultivating the habits in your life that will alleviate your pain. By the end of this book, you will see that not just one thing is responsible for your pain. Your pain is as unique as you are.

Reversing Pain and Weight Gain

What if you could eliminate your pain and shed those additional pounds in the process? What if you could actually start to *feel better*? In *Heal Your Pain Now*, I'll show you how to regain control of your health by breaking the cycle of persistent pain and resistant weight loss. In *Heal Your Pain Now*, you'll discover:

- How to lose 7 to 10 pounds in only 3 weeks
- What is missing from your diet, what to add back into your diet, and how it can help alleviate pain and resistant weight loss
- How to optimize your nutrition with therapeutic and anti-inflammatory foods (Hint: almonds, broccoli, wild salmon, and spinach are a few.)
- The key concepts of a good physical therapy and exercise program
- How to overcome Sedentary Syndrome
- How to burn the most fat in the shortest amount of time
- That quite often "pain is in your brain" and not in your body
- Cognitive retraining exercises to unlearn your pain
- Why your emotions can perpetuate pain
- Meal plans, shopping lists, and recipes to support you throughout the Healing Pain Program

You *can* live a healthy, pain-free, and active life by following the principles of the Healing Pain Program. If you struggle with chronic pain and are overweight, stressed out, fatigued, and depressed, the Healing Pain Program provides the concrete solutions so that you can finally shed the weight, alleviate the pain, and lead an active and fulfilling life.

The Beginning of the End for Pain

The Healing Pain Program is designed to reset your brain and body for a pain-free life. I recommend you read all chapters in sequence to learn as much as you can about your pain and how to heal it. If you have lived with persistent pain, you will benefit most from engaging with each chapter and applying the lessons learned to your life. Set aside time each day to complete some reading—make notes on the pages if needed! This is a guide to help you heal, move again, and live pain-free. Enlist a friend or family member to support you or read the book together. Working with a support group will help you, and others can hold you accountable to keep you on track. You can join my healing pain support group by visiting www.drjoetatta.com/group.

The Healing Pain Program will accelerate your ability to heal. I have spent my entire career treating people who are in pain. They now once again lead fulfilled and active lives and enjoy living without pain. The benefits you will receive from implementing the changes will not only optimize your health but also reduce your pain *and* the number on the scale. Your opportunity to make the transformation and to take back your life and health is here. Your time is now. It is an honor to take this journey with you, and I look forward to hearing your story of pain and how you reset your brain and body for a pain-free life!

Part I

Beginning the Healing Pain Program

1

RECOGNIZE THE
NEED FOR A RESTART

That you are reading this book suggests you have already realized that it's time for a change. Living day in and day out with persistent pain is *not* a lifestyle. Chances are you were not born this way. Pain was not a constant in your life and extra weight was not a problem. You were probably born healthy, explored your environment, moved about with ease as a child, and never thought about physical limitations.

Unfortunately, this may no longer be how you feel or who you are. You have lost your identity and self, due to pain. If you are like most, you have seen the numbers on the scale progressively increase and felt your clothes become tighter. It has become more difficult to move and negotiate through daily life. As the number on the scale has risen, so has your pain scale number. Some days it's a 5/10, and others it's a 9/10, and you can barely function. Pain has permeated every facet of your life. Basic activities around the home are more difficult, exercise is minimal and intimidating, friendships are less connected, and the amount of time it takes to perform routine tasks is time consuming and energy draining. You're not alone. In fact, in many ways you are part of the majority. When did the United States become a nation in pain?

Many people have struggled with persistent pain for years. We are rapidly becoming aware of the global impact on our health and ability, and we now know that certain "comorbidities" or conditions become additional problems for the overweight and obese. Persistent pain and the multitude of pain-type syndromes are highly correlated with obesity. Reducing your weight is an important factor and often the fastest way to alleviating your pain.

Do you really have to live in pain and lose the ability to be physically active or perform daily activities? Do you have to gain weight just because you've turned thirty, forty, or fifty? No. Absolutely not! You do *not* have to live your life in pain and overweight. Don't believe the myth that *as you get older, you will get heavier and everything will hurt.* There is no reason you shouldn't be able to walk up a flight of stairs, lift groceries, or squat down to play with your child. Belly fat is not a badge of honor for entering middle age. This myth is completely false, and if you follow the suggestions and protocols of the Healing Pain Program as outlined in this book, you can live a vital and fit life well into your later years. This chapter will explore the intrinsic link between pain and weight gain and how you can conquer both, using an integrated functional medicine approach that simultaneously focuses on nutrition, movement, and mind training. It's time to end the struggle and restart your life!

You can benefit from this book if . . .

- You need a guide to recover from chronic disease.
- You have a painful inflammatory condition.
- You have an autoimmune condition.
- You live with persistent pain.
- You need to lose weight.
- You have trouble performing basic daily activities.
- You need to transform your health and stay healthy!

The Growth of Obesity

Obesity is a condition whereby excessive fat tissue accumulates and is usually diagnosed by using weight and height to calculate body mass index, or BMI. A person can have a low, normal, overweight, or obese BMI. A BMI greater than 40 is considered morbidly obese. About 3.5 percent of Americans are morbidly obese, which does not sound like a high number until you realize that it translates to about 12.5 million people. It's as if every person who lives in New York City, Boston, and Philadelphia is morbidly obese.

According to the World Health Organization (WHO), 39 percent of adults globally are overweight and 13 percent are obese. In the United States, the rates of obesity are known to exceed those in the rest of the world, with 69 percent of Americans overweight and 35 percent obese. Obesity is also a significant risk factor for a host of medical problems, including diabetes, cancer, heart disease and stroke, high blood pressure, osteoarthritis, respiratory problems, and mood disorders. All this extra weight is a leading reason why people live with persistent pain.

Abdominal Obesity or Central Obesity

Central obesity is characterized as excessive abdominal fat around the stomach, abdomen, and back. Fat accumulation in this part of the body has a negative impact on health. Obesity remains a critical population health concern because of its effects on pain, disease, disability, and health-care costs.

Pain and Suffering

Pain is associated with a wide range of injury and disease, and can be a disease by itself. Millions suffer with chronic pain each day, and the effects of pain place a tremendous financial burden on their nation in health-care costs and lost worker productivity, as well as the emotional and financial burden it places on patients, families, and communities. People often miss work because of back pain, headaches, arthritis, and other musculoskeletal conditions. Adults with persistent pain are more likely to have poorer health, rely on health care, and suffer from greater disability than those with less pain.

Pain has become a problem for almost every facet of the US population, including children and baby boomers—the fastest growing segment of the population. Each day, ten thousand boomers turn sixty-five years old, adding to our growing elderly population. Persistent pain does increase with age, particularly joint pain and painful neuralgias. People are as desperate for solutions to their pain as they are to their weight gain. The following chart depicts the number of chronic pain sufferers compared to other major health conditions.

Condition	Number of People Suffering
Chronic pain	~100 million Americans
Diabetes	~25 million Americans
Cardiovascular disease	~23 million Americans
Cancer	~12 million Americans

Double Trouble: Obesity and Pain

There is a definitive link between excess weight and painful conditions, such as osteoarthritis, spinal and joint pain, autoimmune disease, diabetes, and metabolic syndrome. It is now clear that mechanical (the body's physical makeup), metabolic (the internal chemical reactions), and psychosocial factors (behavior, environment, and lifestyle) all have significant contributing and lasting effects on this chronic health problem. The lifestyle you lead directly impacts your ability to live healthy or live in pain. According to the Arthritis Foundation, losing 15 pounds may decrease knee pain by 50 percent. Just as weight gain causes more pain, weight loss reduces pain. *You have the power to increase or decrease your pain*—and it's tied directly to your weight.

There is no doubt that as we have gained weight, so, too, have we carried more pain. Studies from the early 1990s point to one in seven people struggling with persistent pain, whereas more recent studies now support a much higher percentage: Almost 25 percent of us live with persistent pain. As our obesity epidemic has risen, so, too, have the levels of pain we carry.

The obesity-pain connection is a serious public health concern for our society. In an article in the *Journal of Epidemiology*, researchers surveyed 1,010,762 people, calculating their BMI (measure of body fat) and asked them the following two questions: "1) Did you experience pain yesterday; and 2) In the last 12 months, have you had any neck or back condition that caused recurring pain, knee or leg condition that caused recurring pain, or other condition that caused recurring pain?" A definitive association between BMI classification and pain emerged.

This study indicated that for each BMI class greater than Low through Normal, a higher probability of pain existed. The authors reported that as BMI increased so did pain, with 20 percent more pain in the Overweight group, 68 percent more in Obese I, 136 percent in Obese II, and 254 percent in Obese III. It's important to note that the sample size of this study was greater than a million people, which is very large; most studies typically involve fewer than one hundred subjects. The data linking persistent pain and extra weight is significant.

Chronic Inflammation:
The Root Cause of Obesity and Pain

I'm here to paint a picture for you of what has been transpiring in your body for years or decades and has led to chronic inflammation—and ultimately keeping you in pain and overweight. Inflammation is actually the root cause of most diseases, and obesity is perhaps the kingpin of inflammatory conditions. Obesity not only causes increased inflammation but also makes it harder to lose weight! This is known as resistant weight loss. People may be in different places on the inflammatory spectrum, according to their lifestyle habits and environment. If you eat an extremely healthy diet, exercise five hours a week, and meditate for ten minutes daily, chances are you don't have signs of chronic inflammation. But if you eat the standard American diet (SAD)—which consists of way too much sugar and processed foods and not enough fruits, vegetables, fiber, healthy fats, vitamins, and minerals; do not exercise; take multiple prescription drugs; and have no weekly self-care routine (and I'm not talking about your hair and nails!), then you undoubtedly have a moderate amount of inflammation in your body. And if this has been the norm for the majority of your life up to and including your fifth decade, then you are probably struggling with one or more of the diseases caused by significant and persistent inflammation.

Living with obesity equals living a proinflammatory life. Gone are the days when we perceived the weight around our midsection as static, dead weight that we simply lugged around. No, sir, belly fat is an active metabolic factory that pumps out inflammatory chemicals all day long, even when you are sleeping! This inflammation in turn leads to chronic activation of your immune system. Proinflammatory cytokines—the chemicals released by your immune cells—and hormones secreted by fat tissue can generate and perpetuate chronic inflammation. Constant inflammation can lead to insulin resistance—also called metabolic syndrome—which is pervasive in our society. Experts estimate that 25 percent of all Americans suffer from insulin resistance. I believe the percentage is much higher among those who struggle with persistent pain.

Continuing on the insulin resistance path leads to type 2 diabetes, and perhaps the fastest way to develop a life of obesity and pain. Diabetes is caused by inefficient insulin hormone use or insufficient production by the body, which affects blood sugar levels. What would a hormone and blood sugar condition have to do with pain? Well, a diet full of empty calories—sugar and refined carbohydrates, all of which convert to sugar—eventually leads to insulin resistance and type 2 diabetes. Chronically high blood sugar (hyperglycemia) will ultimately lead to low levels of insulin, because your pancreas cannot keep up with the demand. Your body will finally lose the battle and fail to produce enough insulin to keep up with the amount of sugar and refined carbohydrates you are consuming. This leaves you daily with toxic levels of blood sugar, insulin resistance, and type 2 diabetes. Among the many problems of chronically high blood sugar is inflammation—and inflammation means pain!

Processed Foods → Inflammation → Weight Gain → Pain

The large dose of blood sugar that accompanies a meal or snack of highly refined carbohydrates (white bread, white rice, French fries, sugar-laden soda, and so on) increases cytokines, the chemical messengers of inflammation. Each time you eat, you have the ability to increase or decrease the amount of inflammation in your body, as well as to influence your pain and waist size! Learning to eat according to the Healing Pain Program will smooth out the after-meal rise in blood sugar and insulin and dampen cytokine production.

> ## Diabesity
>
> The continuum of health problems, ranging from mild insulin resistance and being overweight to obesity and diabetes

Diabetics also develop a condition known as peripheral neuropathy. It is caused by nerve damage, which can cause pain and limit activity. According to the US Department of Health and Human Services, between 60 and 70 percent of people with diabetes have some form of neuropathy. Diabetes destroys not only the musculoskeletal system but also the nervous system—the two most important systems with regard to pain.

> ## Chronic Inflammatory Conditions Causing Pain and Weight Gain
>
> - Obesity
> - Osteoarthritis
> - Spinal and joint pain
> - Certain cancers
> - Rheumatoid arthritis
> - Lupus
> - Adrenal fatigue
> - Thyroiditis
> - Multiple sclerosis
> - Parkinson's disease
> - Type 2 diabetes
> - Irritable bowel syndrome
> - Mood disorders (depression, anxiety)
> - Cardiovascular disease

All this leads to a nation that is overweight, in pain, and losing its physical vitality. Basic daily activities have now become a challenge for many in the United States, due to the pain and weight gain they struggle with on a daily basis:

- 17.2 million adults are unable or find it difficult to walk a quarter-mile.
- 35.2 million adults have some physical functioning difficulty.
- 75.4 adults aged 18 and older have at least one daily activity limitation or multiple activity limitations.

This is no way to live. Eliminating chronic inflammation through diet and activity can reduce your weight and pain.

Metabolic Syndrome = Three or More of the Following:

Abdominal obesity
(measured by waist circumference):   men > 40 inches; women >35 inches
Triglycerides: > 150 mg/dL or on lipid-lowering drugs
Low HDL: men < 40 mg/dL; women <50 mg/dL
Blood pressure: > 130/85 mmHg or on antihypertensive
                                     medication
Fasting glucose: > 100 mg/dL

Factors of a Proinflammatory Lifestyle

- Processed foods high in sugar suppress the immune system.
- Lack of fiber in diet (Fiber helps pull toxins from the gut and eliminate them.)
- Lack of movement/exercise fosters excess adipose tissue, which is proinflammatory. (Exercise helps increase and maintain lean muscle mass, which improves insulin sensitivity and burns fat.)
- Vitamin and mineral deficiencies, especially vitamin D
- Toxin exposure
- Emotional stress/toxic relationships
- Lack of joy and purpose
- Leaky gut (dysbiosis)
- Food allergens
- Lack of phytonutrients

The Healing Pain Program

You already know that eating fried food is bad for your body, too much stress causes high blood pressure, and sitting in front of the television for hours instead of being active is a recipe for disaster. The three pillars of chronic disease include a sedentary lifestyle, poor nutrition, and depression. They systematically wear you down day by day, slowly but steadily damaging your health and eroding your body. Unfortunately, I've seen that it often takes a health crisis for a patient to change his or her lifestyle. Too many people rely on food for comfort, and the thought of losing a significant amount of weight can seem inconceivable and overwhelming—especially to someone in serious pain. That you are reading this book suggests you are probably tired of being in pain, recognize the need for a restart, and know that it's time to try something different. Health transformations are often challenging, but they can also be exciting and rewarding as you begin to see real results. And hopefully by now you can see the clear link between added weight and pain and understand that if you start to reduce your weight, it will have a positive effect on your pain.

I often have patients who may be working hard on the physical aspect of their program, but it's not until they begin to alter their diet that they finally achieve results. Margaret struggled with on-again, off-again lower back pain for nearly a decade. Like many people with lower back pain, she had seen her share of chiropractors, physical therapists, and massage therapists. She was mostly sedentary and did not have a regular exercise routine, but she did have a list of exercises she performed for her back three times a week. I adjusted her lower back program to include more extension-based exercises, since she spent most of her day sitting. She was quick to incorporate the exercise into her life but still had little relief if she was not actually moving. Margaret was also overweight and survived on a diet of coffee and a croissant in the morning, processed convenience food for lunch, and a dinner loaded with starchy carbohydrates. After about a month of initiating a few of the changes in "Core Nutritional Healing" (Chapter 5), her lower back pain improved and she lost 7 pounds. As the weight and pain began to decrease, her ambition for more exercise followed and she joined a gym.

Real pain care requires an integrative solution that recognizes the importance of what you put into your body, how you move your body, and the power of your mind to heal your body. The Healing Pain Program takes a functional medicine approach that incorporates nutrition, movement, and mind-set, because people who are in pain are in a unique situation that requires a special set of strategies. As you're transforming your diet, you will also be learning the right ways to move your body, and how your thoughts and emotions can impact your success. It's hard to believe that changing your diet, exercise, and thoughts can make a real difference in a short amount of time. But I'm here to tell you that it absolutely can. If you follow my program, you will begin to lose weight quickly—many people lose 10 pounds within the first three weeks. And as you start to lose weight and lessen the inflammation in your body, you will notice that your pain decreases as well and you really do start to feel better.

The Healing Pain Diet Program

Nutrition should be the first intervention for solving your persistent pain. My nutritional plan will help you eliminate the foods that keep you in pain and pack on the pounds, by focusing on healthy, anti-inflammatory foods that promote repair, healing, energy, and recovery. There are three phases to the Healing Pain Diet Program: core nutritional healing, gut healing, and ketogenic healing. Many people only need to complete the first two phases of the program to achieve real results.

During core nutritional healing (see Chapter 5), you will cut out all processed foods and incorporate more omega-3 fatty acids into your meals, as they will help curb the inflammatory process in your joints and body. You will also consume phytonutrient dense foods in a rainbow of colors, because these therapeutic foods have many healing properties that will have an impact on your pain and your ability to lose weight.

After this phase, you will begin gut healing (see Chapter 6), by eliminating the food culprits that are known to cause inflammation and pain, such as gluten, GMOs (genetically modified organisms, especially those found in soy and corn), sugar, dairy, and eggs. Once you eliminate these foods, you will notice a major improvement in your pain, lose additional weight, have more energy, and sleep better.

After four weeks, if your body is weight-loss resistant and pain is still persistent, you will move toward ketogenic healing (see Chapter 7), where you consume more fat and eliminate all grains, legumes, and starchy carbs. Ketogenic healing will create a state that not only burns fat but will also have a positive effect on your brain and pain.

The Healing Pain Movement Program

Because of their musculoskeletal imbalances and pain, many people have forgotten how to move and don't move regularly during the day. I want you to relearn how to move, and I will help your movement become easy, effortless, smooth, coordinated, and strong. The Healing Pain Movement Program will explain what you should be doing and why you should be doing it. It will not only get your body moving again but also burn that unwanted fat. You will start with the basics and gradually increase your fitness level.

In Chapter 8, "Return to Movement," we will explore the new paradigm of what I call Sedentary Syndrome, which encompasses: central obesity (belly fat), poor posture, sarcopenia (muscle loss), joint failure, and daily life challenges, such as walking up stairs, squatting, or lifting. You will assess your physical status with a series of tests/quizzes and a ten-step physical exam. These exercises constitute a general mobility program that you can begin at home, and they will engage various parts of your body to get it moving again.

Once you are more comfortable with general movement, the challenge is to make an effort to continue moving your body for health, healing, and weight loss. This is where strength or resistance training becomes so important, and in Chapter 9, "Strengthen and Revitalize," we will review the science of strength training and why it's more important than cardiovascular/endurance exercise. In this section, I will provide resistance training guidelines and exercises, so that you can follow a program at least two days per week. The five key exercises include pushing, pulling, squatting, lunging, and core work.

After you have a base of strength and functional movement, the intensity of your workouts can increase. High-intensity interval training (HIIT) is the most efficient form of exercise and often requires just seven minutes. HIIT involves alternating short intervals of high-intensity exercise with short intervals of rest in between. You will lose fat not muscle and achieve more weight-loss progress in fifteen minutes than an hour spent on the treadmill beating your body into submission.

The Healing Pain Mind Program

Finally, as part of my integrative approach, I'll teach you how to train your brain to stop your pain in the Healing Pain Mind Program, by providing a clear set of prescriptive strategies to help eradicate the fear, avoidance, and negative thought patterns that may be inhibiting your recovery. In Chapter 10, "Use Your Brain, Stop Your Pain," you will learn what's really happening to your brain when you are in pain. Many elements, such as fear, avoidance, anxiety, memories, thoughts, movements, sensations, and much more, can magnify your pain experience. For example, if you injure your back while lifting something and you're in a negative state of mind, your brain can actually perceive that pain as worse than it is. So, what's the good news? You can actually train your brain to shut off pain.

The brain matters. And, in fact, the reason so many other pain-management programs fail is that this crucial element has been left out of the process. The Healing Pain Mind Program will provide you with concrete strategies for using your brain to your advantage to overcome your pain. You'll learn such techniques as graded motor imagery, visualization, forgiveness, acceptance and commitment therapy, meditation, and healing intentions to help you transform your thought patterns from a negative space to a positive one. You will be amazed by how much a shift in focus can impact your pain level. Learning about how pain is created can actually change your brain chemistry.

Don't become another pain statistic—you know you are ready for a restart. The Healing Pain Program can help you finally eliminate your pain—and get your weight under control. The Healing Pain Program will encompass nutrition, movement, and mind-set for a more integrated approach to your health.

Dr. Joe's Pain Relief Reminders

- Persistent pain and the multitude of pain-related syndromes are highly correlated with obesity.
- Nutrition and weight loss are the fastest method for alleviating your pain.
- You can reduce chronic inflammation with a healthy diet and exercise.
- Don't forget about your brain's influence on your pain.

2

WHY OTHER TREATMENTS MAY HAVE FAILED YOU

We live in a world where the medical technology is advancing rapidly, and we can now see and detect health issues like never before. This is especially helpful in diagnosing diseases, such as cancer, or in cases of trauma where an image can indicate the best course of treatment and swiftest care. Our medical centers are designed around diagnosing and testing, but this primarily applies to acute medical situations. We have the best acute-care, disease-model medical system in the world, but we lack a *true* health-care system. A true health-care system would be designed to teach people how to live a vital life. Your problem is likely not acute but chronic. You have struggled with persistent pain for years, and truthfully, fancy tests and imaging are not really going to serve you. In fact, they may very well harm you . . . and your wallet!

Your health is perhaps the most important part of your life and your launching point to a successful existence. Whether you strive to be an athlete, a supermom, or a CEO, knowing the status of your health and where to begin your transformation is vital. Tests have their place and are needed, but no one teaches us how to stay healthy—and that includes how to prevent pain. The truth is the *real* tests needed to identify your current health status are simple, easy, and inexpensive.

How We Currently Treat Pain

Before we delve into the specifics of your self-assessment in Chapter 4, I want to explore our current health-care and pain-management situation to illustrate why the system likely isn't working for you and is instead costing you unnecessary money. At present many doctors from different specialties or subspecialties, ranging from neurosurgery, neurology, orthopedics, psychology, anesthesiology, psychiatry, chiropractic, and physical therapy, are involved in the care of pain patients. We have a highly specialized medical system that primarily uses expensive tests, pharmaceuticals, and surgery to address pain. There is a bias for surgeons to operate, anesthesiologists to perform pain procedures, physical therapists to emphasize movement, and psychologists to use cognitive behavioral modification techniques. Each treatment represents a particular doctor's education and training.

In acute situations, our existing system is perhaps the best in the world. However, imaging studies, surgeries, and medications have not changed the persistence of our pain. The approaches we are currently using simply don't work. We do not have a common *blueprint* for how to treat persistent pain. The medical system can be a maze of practitioners for a patient to negotiate through trial and error as well as a financial burden. According to a survey, 63 percent of pain sufferers see their family doctor for help, and 40 percent see a specialist, such as an orthopedist. A large proportion of people consult more than one practitioner in the medical community.

Expensive Testing ≠ Better Care

In many ways our traditional health-care system has failed those who are living with chronic pain. Pain (and obesity) are on the rise globally; government, private insurers, and world health organizations are unprepared for the associated costs of disability, which has the potential to greatly impact economies worldwide. How can you lose weight when you are suffering from "chronic" diseases, such as fibromyalgia, diabetes, or arthritis? We have an abundance of conditions and diagnostic labels. But where is the plan to help people recover?

We function in a system that rewards the use of prescription medication, expensive diagnostic images, and procedures instead of education, inspiration, and conservative treatment. People often come to a physical therapist last—although more and more are choosing to see a physical therapist first. If you did not choose physical therapy first, you have probably had a long journey through the medical system to arrive at our door. You may have started at your internist, who performed a general physical exam, checking blood pressure, heart rate, and respiration, and possibly ran some blood work. Maybe he or she looked at the basic range of motion of one joint, if you're lucky. Then your internist referred you on to a "specialist," which could include any number of physicians—orthopedists, physiatrists, rheumatologists, and pain management doctors are typically next in line. They likely performed more tests. Here is a short list of the many tests you may have been forced to undergo:

- X-rays
- MRIs
- CT scans
- Bone density scan (a.k.a. DXA or bone densitometry)
- Fluoroscopy
- Ultrasound
- EMG and nerve conduction studies
- Arthroscopy
- Basic blood work

These tests certainly serve their place, especially with regard to trauma, and I'm not against them in theory or completely. But we now have plenty of research that directs us away from testing for *chronic* conditions. So, if you don't have an acute injury from a recent car accident but instead suffer from chronic back pain that you've had for years, a battery of tests may not be the best place to begin.

Imaging Abnormalities Are Common in Everyone

Although tests can be helpful in acute situations, they can actually do more harm than good when it comes to understanding, identifying, and solving chronic pain. Low back pain is perhaps the best example. Low back pain is the leading cause of activity limitation and work absence throughout the world, and chronic low back pain—pain lasting more than three months—is rapidly increasing. Many patients with low back pain receive routine spinal imaging, such as lumbar radiography (X-ray), computed tomography (CT scan), or magnetic resonance imaging (MRI). Imaging studies, however, have frequent false positive and negative results and are often poor indicators of what is really causing your pain. In short, they are only a picture. The American College of Physicians and the American Pain Society currently recommend using imaging only for severe or progressive neurological deficits or where a serious underlying condition or disease is suspected. Red flags include a history of cancer, unexplained weight loss, recent infection, loss of bowel control, urinary retention, or loss of strength. They also stated that routine imaging does not result in clinical benefit and may lead to harm! Imaging can subject the body to unnecessary radiation as well as lead to additional tests, follow-up, and referrals and may result in an invasive procedure of limited or questionable benefit.

Many abnormalities detected with advanced imaging are so common in healthy, uninjured people that they could be viewed as normal signs of aging. In a cross-sectional study in the *Journal of Bone & Joint Surgery,* 36 percent of healthy participants aged sixty or older had a herniated disc, 21 percent had spinal stenosis, and more than 90 percent had a degenerated or bulging disk! For many of us, when it comes to these abnormalities, it's like having gray hair—we all have some but it doesn't mean we are old and inactive. In fact, most lumbar imaging abnormalities are common in people *without* low back pain and are poorly correlated with symptoms. Disk herniations, degenerative disk disease, spondylosis, and arthritis of the spine occur in everyone's back and are quite frankly a normal part of aging. The tests are excellent at detecting smaller and smaller abnormalities, but poorly correlate with pain. Before you undergo a battery of tests and spend your time and hard-earned money, it is important to understand that the presence of imaging abnormalities does not mean that those abnormalities are responsible for symptoms. Imaging is poorly correlated with pain.

Low back pain is perhaps the most widely researched part of the body in terms of how we assess and treat pain and dysfunction. However, each day we are discovering similar findings for all joints of the body, including the cervical spine, shoulder, and knee. We are learning that your pain, weight, thoughts, and function are the most important factors to assess—and might even be more important than imaging or radiographic finding. We are finding conservative treatment works just as well or better than invasive procedures.

An abnormal reading on an imaging study does not necessarily reveal the root cause of your pain. Instead, it may lead to an expensive and unnecessary procedure that won't result in any better healing than less invasive approaches. Physical therapy may be an effective alternative for patients who would like to avoid surgery.

Imaging Tests for Lower Back Pain

The problem: Getting an X-ray, CT scan, or MRI can seem like a good idea. But back pain usually subsides in about a month, with or without testing. Back-pain sufferers in a 2010 study who had an MRI within the first month didn't recover any faster than those who didn't have the test—but they were eight times as likely to have surgery and had a fivefold increase in medical costs.

The risks: One study projected 1,200 new cancer cases based on the 2.2 million CT scans performed for lower back pain in the United States in 2007. CT scans and X-rays of the lower back are especially worrisome for men and women of childbearing age, because they can expose testicles and ovaries to substantial radiation. Finally, the tests often reveal abnormalities that are unrelated to the pain but can cause fear, anxiety, and lead to additional treatments, including surgery.

The costs: An X-ray of the lower back typically ranges from $200 to $285; an MRI, from $875 to $1,225; and a CT scan, from $1,080 to $1,520. Imaging accounts for a big chunk of the billions Americans spend as they search for the cause of their pain each year.

When to consider the tests: When conservative treatment, such as physical therapy, exercise, alternative medicine, nutrition, and cognitive behavioral approaches, have failed or you have a history of cancer or other disease.

An Overdose of Opioids

The United States is in the midst of an epidemic of prescription and illicit opioid overdose deaths, which killed more than twenty-eight thousand people in 2014 alone. *Every day, more than forty Americans die from prescription opioid overdoses.* Opioid pain medication is the third most common drug prescribed after medication for depression (those, too, are often prescribed for pain!). As I was writing this book, the Obama administration petitioned Congress for 1 billion dollars to combat the epidemic of pain and addiction. Prescription narcotics for pain relief are on the rise, leading to abuse and frequently the gateway to heroin addiction. In March 2016 the Centers for Disease Control and Prevention (CDC) published its "Guidelines for Prescribing Opioids for Chronic Pain." The CDC guidelines were created in response to growing rates of opioid use disorder and opioid overdose, a problem fueled by ever-increasing rates of opioid prescriptions written by primary care providers. In 2012, health-care providers wrote 259 million prescriptions for opioid pain medication, enough for every adult in the United States to have a bottle of pills. The new guidelines published by the CDC were groundbreaking and for the first time recommended integrative lifestyle interventions. The recommendations stated:

- Nonpharmacologic therapy and nonopioid pharmacologic therapy are preferred for chronic pain.
- Exercise therapy, nutrition, and cognitive behavioral interventions—often in combination—are preferred for treating chronic pain.

Nearly one third of all US adults are suffering from chronic pain, and 5 percent of them are prescribed an opioid to help cope with the pain. This was almost unheard of until the 1990s. Before then, the only patients receiving opioid treatments were cancer patients or those with acute traumatic pain. As we know, research is an ongoing process, and during the 1990s, studies revealed that all different types of pain were being undertreated.

As a result of those studies, more focus was placed on pain education and advocacy, which led directly to an increase in more doctors prescribing opioids for patients with chronic, but nonterminal, pain. Since 1997, the volume of opioids prescribed in this country has risen by 600 percent. That percentage is astounding, especially when you consider that the number of unintentional lethal overdoses from prescribed opioids has increased right along with it, up to around 350 percent.

Now studies show that nonterminal patients who take opioids for pain relief actually have a lower quality of life and higher rate of depression. In a survey conducted for the American Pain Foundation of people currently using an opioid to treat their pain, 77 percent of respondents reported feeling depressed. Pain sufferers also have decreased energy levels and difficulty sleeping. That same survey revealed that more than half felt they had little or no control over their pain. Even using a small dose of opioids each day can ultimately lower a patient's pain threshold, which is not the direction you want to go in if you are suffering from persistent pain.

Part of the problem with painkillers is that they are often abused, create dependence, and can be addictive. After marijuana, prescription drugs are the most abused drugs in the United States. Even adults over age fifty have used prescription drugs nonmedically, and substance abuse treatment for this age group has risen dramatically in recent years. Deaths from an overdose of opioid pain relievers now exceed deaths from heroin or cocaine abuse. In an alarming new study on prescription drug overdoses referenced in *PT in Motion* magazine, it was discovered that more than 90 percent of people who survived an overdose were actually able to get another prescription for the very same drug after their overdose, often from the same physician. The study suggests a surprising lack of communication between doctors and their patients, a strong imperative for doctors to carefully monitor patients who use opioids, and the necessity of alternative treatments for chronic pain, such as physical therapy and mental health initiatives. Clearly, we have to find a better way to manage pain. Patients deserve safe and effective treatments.

A Functional Approach:
How We *Should* Treat Pain

Functional medicine views the entire body as one integrated system and does not focus on treating symptoms but instead unearthing the root cause of what is preventing health. You treat the entire individual—mind and body. The basis of a functional medicine approach often begins with healing the gut first, as this is where 70 percent of your immune system lives. Through healing your gut, you will optimize your immune system and decrease inflammation—also decreasing pain and your weight! (We'll examine the gut in more detail in Chapter 6.) Functional medicine relies on nutrition, real food, and supplements to begin the healing process and often integrates other tools for healing. It provides a powerful new model to replace the outdated and ineffective acute-care models carried forward from the twentieth century. It enables health professionals to practice proactive, preventative, personalized medicine and empowers patients to take an active role in their own health.

Chronic pain and obesity are two areas where functional medicine can make a significant impact, as both require an integrated approach to effectively remedy them. As you know, treating your persistent pain with a drug has not relieved your symptoms. Functional medicine may utilize traditional medicine when needed; however, it relies on strategies to enhance your body's own innate ability to heal. In both the acute and chronic phases of pain, the use of physical therapy coupled with alternative treatments, including dry needling, acupuncture, nutrition, supplementation, herbal therapy, and mind-body techniques, can be useful. Multiple therapies are often best. For example, in the acute phase, pain management with drugs may be needed; however, in the chronic phase, using prescription painkillers is inefficient and does not lead to improved functional outcomes. The Healing Pain Program delivers an integrative, functional medicine approach to healing, centered on nutrition, movement, and the brain, and invites you to be an active participant in your recovery, by learning the strategies you need to heal.

Too many people are struggling with persistent pain, and the time is now to help them. Change is a challenge for both the practitioners and patients, but most especially for someone in pain. And many of the readily available pills and high-tech procedures don't work for those in pain. We need to prescribe optimal nutrition and movement strategies, along with education centered on coaching and behavioral changes, if we want to reverse the escalating trend of pain. Currently, most clinicians practice a single modality, and the US health-care system keeps its population in silos based on payment and scope of practice battles. *Heal Your Pain Now* is designed to provide you with the integrative strategies necessary to overcome persistent pain. With the right program, we can reverse the trend and help people to find relief for their symptoms. It's time to stop placing so much emphasis on diagnostic imaging, prescription drugs, and invasive surgery, and to instead adopt a more integrative, conservative, mind-body approach to relieving pain with the right nutritional plan, movement, and brain retraining.

Dr. Joe's Pain Relief Reminders

- Opioids are not the answer.
- Expensive tests and imaging procedures do not lead to better health, but to fear and bankruptcy.
- Most people *without* persistent pain also have imaging abnormalities.
- The Healing Pain Program offers an integrative, functional medicine approach that incorporates nutrition, movement, and mind-set to alleviate your pain.

3

YOUR BRAIN IN PAIN

What if I told you that there is another reason you are in pain, and it doesn't have to do with diet and exercise? What if it requires no math, no measuring calories, no worrying about exercise or the structure and function of your joints? There is an explanation for your pain that practically no one speaks about: your brain. We have yet to develop a fancy, expensive test to diagnose it, but your brain is often the real cause of your persistent pain.

This is an essential chapter in your recovery process, and we need to address it before we talk about the specifics of nutrition and exercise—which are also extremely important. Before you begin the Healing Pain Program, you need to fully understand exactly how your body and brain function. Those who are most successful at breaking the persistent pain cycle are those who educate themselves and then use that education as the fuel to feed their health transformation, with the most information possible. The best program in the world isn't going to work if fear is holding you back from moving your body. Taking control, educating yourself, and breaking through your fear will help you overcome your obstacles. Your brain is literally causing the pain you struggle with every day!

How Your Body Heals

Our body has an innate ability to heal itself. Through evolution we have developed a highly specialized and evolved mechanism for healing. Many of us are aware of our immune system as the part responsible for fighting infection, bacteria, or disease. Our immune system also plays a pivotal role in healing from injury and repairing tissue. If you have ever pulled a muscle, strained a ligament, or broken a bone, your immune system stepped in and healed you.

The classical signs of an acute injury include pain, heat, redness, swelling, and loss of function. You may have experienced these symptoms if you sprained an ankle or caught your finger in a door. The injury swells, turns red, feels hot, and all of these sensations combined cause you to temporarily lose function of a particular part of your body. These are the hallmarks of normal inflammation. The inflammatory process is necessary for healing to occur in the body and follows a predictable path, as long as you are healthy and well.

Injuries heal at different rates, depending on the type of tissue, severity of the injury, and the health of your immune system, environment, diet, and stress level. Soft tissues are most commonly injured and consist of basically every tissue except bone. This includes muscles, ligaments, tendons, joint capsules, disks, nerves, and fascia. A strained muscle often heals in a matter of days, due to its rich blood supply, which brings healthy immune cells to the area for healing and repair. The richer the blood supply to a particular part of your body, the faster an injury will generally heal. Many of us have had fractured bones and know that in approximately six to eight weeks, a fracture will heal.

The Phases of Healing

There are three phases to healing: inflammation, repair, and remodeling. It's helpful to know how each of these stages work so that you better understand why they are important and how they provide your body with exactly what it needs at different times in your recovery process. I also think it's beneficial to fully comprehend how the body

The Three Phases of Healing

1. **Inflammation:** 3–7 days
2. **Repair:** 2–6 weeks
3. **Remodeling:** 3–6 months

operates to heal itself and how long it takes, so that you can see why the pain can be generated by your brain and not your tissues after a certain period of time has elapsed.

Inflammation typically lasts for *three to seven days,* as the body initiates the healing process after an injury. Inflammation is a necessary part of healing and is the phase where pain, redness, and swelling are most prevalent, as your body's immune system releases protein messengers called cytokines that begin the inflammatory process. During this phase, the tissues swell, causing more pain and discomfort to the injured area. Your body's aim at this point is to protect your injury from further damage.

Repair is the second phase of healing. Once the old, injured tissue has been cleared out, your body will begin to repair or replace the torn, strained, or fractured tissue. It does this by laying down new collagen in place of the old, essentially regenerating the tissue you have lost through damage or injury.

The third phase, remodeling, begins as your body stops producing new collagen. Remodeling molds the new tissue so that it resembles the tissue that was injured as closely as possible. The new collagen created during the repair phase may be inelastic or stiff, so it's important to perform certain movements or exercise to make the new tissue nice and pliable and strong. Unfortunately, this is the stage where most people get stuck. Their pain is decreasing, but they may have lingering stiffness, making them fearful to move the injured area. Unless the tissues are reeducated to move, the problem will persist, worsen, or relapse. Therefore, this stage involves retraining joints, muscles, ligaments, and tendons so they can move again and often includes physical therapy. Once functional movement returns to preinjury level, healing is considered complete.

If pain continues beyond three months, it is now considered to be chronic or persistent pain. Here is where your first breakthrough will begin! The question you should be asking yourself right now is: *If the phases of healing are predictable, and tissue heals in three months, why do I still have pain?* One possibility is that you do not have a strong immune system, you have an autoimmune disease, or the environment in or around your body is not optimal for healing, which puts you in a state of chronic inflammation. Chronic inflammation will mean persistent pain. Poor lifestyle choices can lead to slow or delayed healing, and I provide strategies for these later in this book.

Many factors can interfere with one or more of the phases of the healing process and lead to impaired healing. Some of them include:

- Poor oxygenation
- Infection
- Age
- Immobility
- Stress
- Diabetes
- Obesity
- Medications
- Alcoholism
- Smoking
- Poor nutrition

Another possibility is that your brain has decided it's in your best interest to remain in pain. This can happen even if you have successfully completed the stages of healing. The ultimate question is: Why has your brain decided to continue producing pain?

Pain Beyond Tissue Healing

After three months, depending on the injury and how fast your body responds, you will have completed the phases of healing, and thus your pain should resolve. You may have been labeled as having chronic pain or have struggled with pain that has persisted well after the healing process has concluded. Delayed healing or an interruption in the healing process is possible if you have a weakened immune system.

If you don't have a weakened immune system, which means tissue has healed, what else can be causing your pain? Remember that your brain is the head honcho over your body. *Your brain ultimately decides whether you experience pain.* In fact, *injury is not needed for pain.* How is that possible? Well, if your brain still perceives that you are in danger then it may generate pain as a warning sign. Let's say, one Saturday afternoon, you decide to clean out the garage rather than play softball. While you are cleaning, you pick up that old 80-pound television the wrong way, and you strain the muscles in your back. Now, remember, muscle has a rich blood supply and heals very rapidly, yet for some reason your back pain persists for months. In fact, it lingers way beyond the three-month period when it should have already healed. What is the cause of your pain in this scenario? You guessed it . . . your brain.

Nociception Not Pain!

Now, when I say your brain is the cause of your pain, many people respond, "Oh, that means I'm crazy and the pain is all in my head," or "Am I imagining these symptoms?" The resounding answer is "no, your pain is very real." This reassures many patients and prevents 911 calls to the shrink! Let's bust a major myth about pain: *Your body has no pain receptors.* What? Yes, you heard me—*there are no pain receptors in your body.* You may be thinking, "No pain receptors? I thought you said my pain was real?" This may come as a shock and be confusing, and you may wonder, "if I have no pain receptors then how do I *feel* pain?" The simple answer is that pain is not something you *feel* but a *decision* your brain makes, based on a variety of inputs and factors.

Pain is both a sensory and an emotional experience. While there are no pain sensors in your body, you do have something called nociceptors. It's their job to carry signals up to your brain, where it is your brain's job to interpret these signals and decide if you are in danger. Your brain's primary purpose is to protect you. Based on current information (as well as past memories), your brain will decide whether pain is needed and serves a purpose. Pain is actually an emotional response to the situation you are in. Yes, *pain is an emotion*, like happiness or sadness. Store this, as we will return to it later. Your brain's only purpose is to decide whether pain serves a function at that particular instant.

An example might help you better understand how your brain is the ultimate decision maker in pain. Let's say you are walking down the street in a high-heeled pair of shoes. You know, the really high sexy heels you wear only to that special event, with that special someone. As you are racing to jump into the limo with Mr. Right, you accidentally twist and sprain your ankle. Instantly, nociceptors (not pain receptors, because we don't have any) send a message to your brain that you have injured your ankle, torn some ligaments, and that you probably won't be dancing the cha-cha at the gala this evening with Mr. Right. Your brain decides in a *microsecond* that you tore a ligament in your ankle, are injured, and that rest and rehab are needed to recover. The pain your brain generates will prevent you from dancing that evening and from any prolonged walking until you begin a program of recovery (time to get to physical therapy). This pain will keep you protected from reinjury and allow healing to begin by modifying your activity appropriately. No running, walking too much, or dancing with Mr. Right tonight.

Now, let's say you are crossing a busy New York City street, while carrying your newborn child in your arms. As you walk across the street, you stumble over a pothole and twist your ankle—the same exact injury as in the previous example. Only in this scenario, you notice the light has changed to green and the traffic is now barreling at you at 40 miles per hour. Your brain must make the decision as to what is more important—your injured ankle *or* getting you and your child safely to the other side of the street. In this example, your brain *decides* a painful ankle won't serve your safety. You will feel no pain as your brain instantly makes the executive decision that pain would prevent you from running. You need to run, because it's necessary to *save your life*.

The injury is identical in both examples. In the first example you have pain, and in the second you do not have pain. Why? The tissue damage will be similar but the circumstance is different. This explains how even with tissue damage, you can have no pain. Your brain's decision to experience pain is completely different due to the circumstance, because it prioritizes the worst danger. Will the woman with the infant start to feel the pain in her ankle once she safely reaches the sidewalk? Yes. But this example illustrates how you can feel no pain, despite having an injury. So, if the mother in the second example did not feel any pain when she clearly had an injury, doesn't it make sense that you might also feel pain when you do not have a physical injury or once your body has actually physically healed?

How Pain Is Created in Your Brain

We have learned more about pain science in the last ten years than we have in the last hundred. Progressive and rapid research from the fields of neuroscience, physical therapy, and psychology have slowly but steadily unearthed the mystery of how the brain is the "head honcho" when it comes to pain. You see, your brain is constantly changing, based on your environment and the input it receives. This concept is known as neuroplasticity, or simply plasticity. The term *neuroplasticity* is derived from the root words *neuron* and *plastic*. A *neuron* refers to the nerve cell and its various parts, such as axon, dendrites, and the small space linking two nerves called the synapse. The word *plastic* means "capable of being molded, sculpted, or modified." Neuroplasticity is your brain's potential to reorganize by creating new neural pathways and adapting as needed. Plasticity was a wonderful finding when it was first discovered, because it informed us that our brain had the potential to learn right into old age, right to the very last day. We now know it is never too late to acquire new abilities, such as a language, dancing, or singing.

As you use your brain to learn additional skills, neurons will grow, sprouting new connections that enable you to grasp the coordination necessary to learn the cha-cha, articulate a new phrase, such as "*¿hola, como estas?*" while on vacation in Mexico, and carry a tune while singing in the shower. We have seen this type of science applied to those who have suffered a traumatic brain injury, where parts of the brain have been severely damaged. Other areas of the brain will take over, and neurons will begin to sprout new connections used for relearning activities that were once automatic. The concept of neuroplasticity— and the ability of the brain to reorganize itself in both structure and function—is truly remarkable. For example, people who are visually impaired can engage their visual cortex for fine sensory discrimination when using their hands. In these situations, neuroplasticity appears to be a positive adaptation to loss of function. With pain, however, plasticity seems to go a bit awry.

While your brain has amazing capabilities for adaptation and growth, it takes into account many different factors when deciding to create a pain response—and all of these signals can have an impact on its decision and interfere with neuroplasticity. For example, during your pain experience, your brain also receives information connected to that experience, such as your thoughts, memories, movements, sensations, emotions, sights, smells, and so on. All of these factors have an influence on your brain's decision to create pain. Essentially, pain is an experience your brain has created based on past experiences, upbringing, cultural influences, thoughts, emotions, your environment, and your current stress level. With persistent pain, these factors are continuing to affect your brain's decision to create pain, and they are interfering with your healing. For example, if you often have negative thoughts or are consumed by fear, anger, and guilt, your brain will continue to create a pain response long after your initial injury.

Understanding neuroplasticity has put an end to the old worldview of pain as simply a sensation transmitted along hard-wired paths up and into the brain. Neuroplasticity occurs in your brain as an attempt by your central nervous system (brain and spinal cord) to adapt to injury in a positive way. But in the case of persistent pain, neuroplasticity can be maladaptive and at times work against those trying to cure themselves from pain. Your brain is a large receiver, kind of like a satellite up in space that is constantly receiving signals. Satellites can receive signals from the numerous cell phone towers below on Earth. It is a satellite's job to receive information from the various places, decipher the information, and then transmit a signal. Your brain is similar to that satellite, because it is constantly receiving information. Nociceptive input sends danger signals from your skin, joints, and muscles to be interpreted by your brain. For example, if you sprain your ankle, information about an injury will be sent to your brain. However, this is far from the only information your brain is receiving and processing. At the same exact time, your brain is also receiving visual input via the optic nerve in your eyes, smell from olfactory nerves in your nose, sound from your auditory nerve, and even taste from your lingual nerve on your tongue.

It does not stop there; your brain is also cross-checking the information it has previously stored to weigh in on its decision. Stored information about pain, in the form of memories, as it relates to past experiences as well as beliefs and cultural influences also significantly contributes to the brain's present decisions. And issues such as stress, anxiety, post-traumatic stress disorder (PTSD), or depression can contribute even more input. Combine all of this data, along with lifestyle factors (nutrition, weight, sleep), and your brain has quite a job on its hands. This matrix of information is considered by the brain and occurs in a millisecond! These are just some of the multitude of factors your brain considers before pain is created. If your brain receives enough danger signals from the variety of inputs it receives, it will trigger the alarm and your brain will create pain. This is why different people have different amounts of pain, even with similar injuries, or why your pain can change from day to day. It can also help explain why pain fluctuates throughout the day, with stress (such as when you argue with a spouse or have a deadline at work) or when fear kicks in (at the dentist!). The brain creates pain based on many factors. How much pain your brain creates is based on how many danger signals it receives from the various inputs as well as how "sensitive" your nervous system has become.

An Oversensitive Nervous System

Central sensitization is a condition of the nervous system that is associated with the development and maintenance of chronic pain. When central sensitization occurs, the nervous system is in a persistent state of high reactivity. This constant state of reactivity will maintain pain even after the initial injury might have healed. How do you know whether your symptoms of pain are due to an oversensitive nervous system? The changes of central sensitization occur after repeated experiences with pain. First, identify whether you have any type of inflammatory or metabolic disorder or disease, such as autoimmunity, diabetes, metabolic syndrome, insulin resistance, heart disease, or other tissue pathology. If you fall into one of these categories, Chapter 6, "Gut Healing," will be your launching point to heal your pain, as well as incorporating regular healthy movement into your life. However, it is important to note that if you have struggled with these diseases for years, resulting in fear of movement, anxiety, or depression, then central sensitization is likely a contributing factor—even with a disease process that can cause tissue destruction.

Recent studies in the *Journal of Rheumatology* have implicated central sensitization in those with rheumatic diseases and autoimmunity, such as multiple sclerosis, autoimmune thyroiditis, rheumatoid arthritis, fibromyalgia, Sjögren's syndrome, and many others. If you do not have inflammation and you are well past the stages of healing (three months), it is likely central sensitization is causing your persistent pain. Increasingly, research is demonstrating how the brain clearly plays a role in many different chronic pain disorders. It can occur with chronic low back pain, chronic neck pain, whiplash injuries, chronic tension headaches, migraine headaches, osteoarthritis, endometriosis, injuries sustained in a motor vehicle accident, and following surgeries. Fibromyalgia, irritable bowel syndrome, pelvic pain, interstitial cystitis, and chronic fatigue syndrome all have central sensitization as a common denominator as well.

Central sensitization has two main characteristics; both involve a heightened sensitivity to pain. The first is *allodynia*, which is when a person experiences pain with things that are normally not painful like a simple touch or massage. In such cases, the sensation of touch travels, of course, through the nervous system. Because the nervous system is in a continual state of heightened sensitivity, the sensation is registered in the brain as painful or uncomfortable, even when it really shouldn't be. The second is *hyperalgesia*, which occurs when an actual painful stimulus is perceived as more painful than it should be. An example might be if someone pinches your arm, which ordinarily would be mildly painful, and it sends you through the roof with pain. Again, the sensation of pain travels through the nervous system, which is in a constant state of high sensitivity, and the pain is registered in the brain as a heightened level of pain. If you are more than three months past an injury (tissue damage) and you are still having persistent pain, there is a good chance your nervous system has become overly sensitive.

Signs Your Nervous System Is Sensitized

- Pain persists beyond three months.
- Pain spreads past the injury site.
- Pain switches sides.
- Pain increases with stress.
- Pain worsens.

- Even minor movement hurts.
- Pain is unpredictable.
- You can link pain to your thoughts, emotions, or feelings.
- Pain is linked with previous trauma (physical or emotional).

Tag, You're in Pain

Your next question should be: "How does the brain create persistent pain?" Well, many parts of the brain are involved in the creation of pain; it's not just one area. Cortical areas of the brain responsible for movement, memory, smell, sight, thoughts, beliefs, emotions, and sensation all play a role in the brain's decision of pain. All of these nerves work together in a network referred to as a neurotag. Each of the "brain cells" for a particular neurotag also participates in other neurotags. (Your brain is efficient—it is always working!) For example, it is very likely that your neurotag for back pain has some cells that are also involved in the neurotag for thinking about the concept of a bulging disk. So, when someone (a doctor or therapist, for instance) mentions a bulging disk, it activates your neurotag for "bulging disk," and it also activates some of the cells for your back pain neurotag. *Therefore, thinking about a budging disk or seeing one on an image will lower your threshold for activation of your back pain neurotag.* Huh? Re-read this a few times, as it crucial. (You can also visit www.drjoetatta .com/neurotag for a free tutorial!) This is a simple explanation for why pain can be modified by so many different inputs.

Under normal circumstances, a painful neurotag is inhibited, meaning it is dormant and not causing any pain. But if you land on a day where you are stressed, sleep deprived, fighting with your spouse, and you happen to see the commercial for the newest back pain surgery or back pain medication, you can unearth a dormant neurotag in your brain. And this is how pain is created even months or years after an injury has healed! And since neurons and neurotags overlap, this process can be imprecise. This is one reason why pain might spread beyond the area of actual tissue damage, move from one area to another, switch sides, or become harder to locate in a specific area.

Another problematic issue that occurs with chronic pain is a lowered threshold for activation of a particular pain neurotag, meaning that it can be activated more easily by a broader array of inputs. Think of a brand-new radio with a very sensitive volume button. You can just tap it, and the volume is alarmingly loud. In the same way, the smallest input can activate the neurotag. This is called sensitization, and it explains why pain that persists might become activated with less and less stimulus. For some people with a high degree of sensitization, just thinking about moving, or the fear they anticipate with moving a particular part of their body, is sufficient to evoke pain.

Hurt Does Not Equal Harm

There is some major good news coming your way now that you have passed through Pain Science 101! You are doing awesome—stay with me on this journey. Even though your nervous system is overly sensitive, the pain you feel does not equal harm. And no harm means that despite the pain you feel, you are not damaging any tissue or structures. We already know that pain can be related to a change in your tissues. Inflammation from a poor diet, belly fat, and pains from a sprained ankle may all result in some degree of damage to the surrounding tissues. You would assume that the larger the degree of tissue damage, the greater degree of pain. So, why is a paper cut on a finger so painful? Why are migraines so debilitating? What we now understand is that the severity of the pain report is not always an accurate indication of the degree of tissue damage. Paper cuts on a finger typically involve only a minor amount of tissue damage, but the degree of your pain is usually quite high. In comparison, some life-threatening cancers can remain undetected for years, as there are no associated symptoms. What is important for you to understand is that pain is a poor indicator of damage, and in many people with chronic pain it occurs without damage.

With persistent pain, the link between pain and actual damage is weak. And as you know from painful neurotags, pain is not especially reliable at informing us about where the real problem is located; it's a moving target! Even if you do have a physically challenging disease or condition, such as arthritis, it does not mean that pain is a signal to stop and not move. Persistent pain is something you can *desensitize* over time and with the right training. And the training you need to overcome persistent pain and a sensitive nervous system begins with retraining your brain and reframing your relationship to pain.

Stress: The Modern-Day Danger Signal

Your brain holds a few functions as its highest priority, especially your safety and survival. Its primary job is to protect you and alert you to any danger, because keeping you safe from danger is the most efficient way of keeping you alive. Our stress response is our body's way of protecting us. It is a complex but lightning-fast coordination of your nervous (brain), endocrine (hormones), cardiovascular (heart/blood vessels), and musculoskeletal (muscles/bones) systems. It was designed to give you a burst of energy needed to run and flee from danger or the courage and strength to stand your ground and fight it. The fight-or-flight mechanism is a wonderfully evolved human system—until it works against you.

If your brain perceives that a physical injury is placing you at risk, it can make the decision to create pain. Pain is your brain's way of protecting you, signaling that something is wrong or threatening you, and informing you that healing is needed. Unfortunately, your brain is extraordinarily adept at noticing even the smallest danger signs—not just physical injuries—so you will need to begin to shift your perception with regard to your persistent pain. Your thoughts alone are enough to cause your brain to perceive a threat and light up your HPA axis (hypothalamic-pituitary-adrenal axis), causing the fight-or-flight response that negatively affects your pain and your health.

In today's world we rarely tap into our fight-or-flight mechanism the way it was designed. When was the last time you were running from a lion or spear fighting with the neighboring tribe? Even though your fight-or-flight mechanism is not as utilized today, it is still highly in tune to sensing danger signals. However, the danger signals you now experience are different and their frequency has changed. Most of these danger signals your brain receives today are not physical but have to do with your thoughts and emotions, such as stress, anxiety, anger, frustration, and fear. The things you think about, emote about, and hear about from other people. And these can occur daily or multiple times a day, depending on your lifestyle.

Your Body's Stress Response

To fully understand how stressful thoughts can cause increased pain, we need to cover the stress response in detail. We are all familiar with the concept of a big roaring lion, but our daily thoughts can cause the same type of stress response. Let's say you are quietly working at your desk, enjoying your monthly project. Suddenly, you hear *bing, bing*! It's your boss e-mailing you, and the subject line reads "REVISED DEADLINE—PROJECT DUE THIS FRIDAY!" It is Wednesday evening, which gives you less than 24 hours to wrap up the project you thought you had an extra week to finish. How are you going to complete it while you have two kids at home, food shopping that you need to do, and the daily commute to endure? Most would agree this would constitute a threat to your body and elicit an immediate stress response. If this were a one-time event, your body would release the hormone adrenaline to increase your heart rate and respiration, thus increasing blood flow and oxygen to tissues. Adrenaline would switch on the large muscles of your legs and arms, preparing for the fight or flight. Generally, pain is not felt during an acute stress response.

When stress becomes frequent or cumulative—or chronic—and you have to deal with a stressful job, traffic, and financial pressures day in and day out, your body will release the hormone cortisol. Cortisol is best known for taking a stressful thought or emotion and turning it into a physical response to that stress. The most important physical response for you? Pain, tightness, and tension. Cortisol has a similar effect as adrenaline, although it is more potent and lasts longer. When released, cortisol will function to increase blood sugar and suppress the immune system. Simply stated, increased cortisol prevents the release of chemicals in the body that cause inflammation. Now, this may seem like a good thing, as many of us have a negative perception of inflammation, but in reality inflammation is necessary for healing and recovering from an injury. In addition to decreased tissue healing, an overabundance of cortisol can lead to lack of sleep, anxiety, and depression, all of which can exacerbate pain and cause weight gain.

With your adrenal glands pumping out cortisol for long periods of time, there are far-reaching effects in multiple systems of your body. Prolonged and elevated cortisol levels will actually lead to muscle wasting, because your body will begin to metabolize its own muscle for a source of energy. (Your muscles store most of your body's protein and glucose.) Essentially, you may find your muscles shrinking and your waist expanding, as the glucose stripped from your muscles now gets stored on your waist. Less muscle and more belly fat is a recipe for more pain. Changes in cortisol have also been linked to decreased bone formation or the breakdown of bone (your body is looking for extra minerals stored in bone). Cortisol dysregulation is associated with weight gain and obesity—yikes!—because your appetite changes, often leading to cravings, especially for sugar and salt. Your breathing also changes, becoming more shallow and irregular, leading to decreased oxygen. The tissues of your body become hypoxic, actually starving for more oxygen. Your mood may fluctuate between melancholy, anxious, or foggy. And your sleep will suffer, as it becomes harder to fall asleep and remain asleep. So, dysregulated cortisol is causing:

- Increased blood sugar
- A breakdown of healthy muscle and bone
- Lowered immunity
- A change in your appetite

- Weight gain
- Poor oxygenation
- Depression and anxiety
- Insomnia

Because of how our body responds to stress by producing cortisol, stress has a strong impact on our ability to heal pain and lose weight. Too much stress leads to too much cortisol, which leads to pain and weight gain.

Long-Term Effects of Cortisol on Various Body Systems

Musculoskeletal	Hormonal	Immune
Muscle imbalances	Weight gain	Decreased immunity
Painful trigger points	Increased appetite	Prolonged inflammation
Poor balance	Tissue changes	Old injuries hurt
Fatigue	Obesity	Body dysmorphia
Osteoporosis	Fertility	Proneness to illness
Muscle wasting		
Mood	**Respiration**	**Sleep**
Depression	Decreased oxygen	No REM sleep
Anxiety	Fatigue	Problems falling asleep
Mood swings	Tightness in neck/chest	Memory problems
Brain fog	Shallow breathing	
Anger/frustration		
Fatigue		

How Cortisol Causes Weight Gain

When your stress and cortisol levels are high, the body actually resists weight loss. Your body thinks times are hard and you might starve, so it stores fat around your midsection. Cortisol tends to take fat from healthier areas, like your hips, and move it to your abdomen, which has more cortisol receptors. In the process, it turns once-healthy peripheral fat into unhealthy visceral fat (the fat in your abdomen that surrounds your organs), which increases inflammation and insulin resistance in the body. The more cortisol, the more belly fat you will have.

Cortisol levels are also affected by changes in your mood. Living a life in pain and with resistant weight loss is often a one-way ticket to depression and anxiety. A more significant and compounding effect is that changes in cortisol have profound effects on your immune system, promoting chronic inflammation. Whereas inflammation is a good thing immediately following an injury, inflammation that sticks around and never goes away is unhealthy. Cytokines are the little chemicals that your immune cells release to begin the inflammatory process. They should be short lived, but stress and a poor diet can promote cytokine production. Increased cytokine production leads to systemic inflammation or inflammation all over the body, keeping tissues chronically inflamed and preventing healing.

Extra fat also adds a painful twist to the vicious cycle because fat in and of itself is inflammatory. Gone are the days where we think of fat as inert tissue hanging over your belt. Fat is metabolically active; it's a factory producing chemicals that affect your hormonal, endocrine, nervous, and musculoskeletal system. Fat keeps pressure on an already stressed out and painful body.

Your Thoughts Can Generate Pain

Psychological and social factors play an important role in causing pain, especially after an injury has healed. Your thoughts, emotions, behaviors, prior experiences, cultural influences, religion, and work can all have an impact on the brain's decision to produce pain. These factors all influence how the brain and nervous system process injury, disease, danger, and recovery. At the heart of your persistent pain lie your thoughts about pain and your experience. The mind and body are not separate, unrelated issues. At the root of your thoughts, two areas need to be discussed: fear and catastrophizing.

Fear and Avoiding Activity

Fear is defined as "a distressing negative sensation caused by an actual or perceived threat." Notice that the definition says an actual *or perceived* threat. This is important, because your perception of an injury or your environment can influence how much pain you feel. Remember, your thoughts can affect your emotions, which can then affect your pain. Fear of movement, fear of exercise, fear of reinjury, and fear of the recovery process can all have an influence on your pain. Fear may develop from uncertainty about how long an injury will take to heal, not understanding your diagnosis, lack of prognosis, and worrying about how your pain may affect your financial and social life. Not knowing the outcome of your situation can instill fear and dampen recovery or prolong pain.

With fear, people begin to avoid certain things that hasten their recovery. Fear avoidance is a model that describes how individuals develop persistent pain as a result of avoiding behaviors based on fear. The fear-avoidance model can also help you understand how you can experience pain even without an actual injury. If you experience discomfort and avoid treatment by using avoidant behavior, a lack of pain increase reinforces your behavior. For example, if you have a knee pain and you avoid physical therapy for fear that movement will worsen your pain, and then your pain doesn't increase for a few weeks, it may encourage you to keep avoiding physical therapy, even though that is what you truly need to heal. Conversely, if you perceive pain as non-threatening or temporary, you will feel less anxious and confront the pain-related situation.

Avoidant behavior is healthy when needed for your injury to heal, such as during the inflammation phase. However, this can become detrimental to your health once your injury has healed. Fear-avoidance behaviors prevent you from engaging in normal daily activities, normal movement, and normal exercise—all of which restricts normal use of your body and weakens it both physically and mentally.

You can refer to the diagram on page 43 for a visual illustration of how this process works. Injury may be the cause of pain; however, many patients develop persistent pain in the absence of an actual injury, revealing that pain is not always connected to injury. If you are struggling with intense emotional issues, such as those centered around family, work, or societal pressures, they may be the root cause

Fearful Thoughts Contributing to Pain

- Certain movements
- Reinjury
- Not being able to work
- Exercise
- Not being able to assist family
- Needles or surgery
- Drugs
- Not being able to have or care for kids
- Not understanding your diagnosis
- Trying and failing
- Medical practitioners or system
- Not being able to have sex/be intimate
- Asking for help
- Losing your job
- Making it worse
- Ending up disabled
- Not healing
- Test findings

of your pain. Emotional overload can generate pain—this is your brain in pain. The thoughts and feelings you have about life events can actually cause pain. If this is you, the pain is not in your tissues!

Pain Catastrophizing

Consider how you feel at this moment or in the recent past. Is your pain so intense that you can't stop thinking about its consequences? Are you worried the diagnosis the doctor wrote on his or her little white prescription pad is a disability sentence that will affect how you move and function for the rest of your life? Are the imaging study results causing you anxiety? Did a practitioner diagnose you with an autoimmune disease and tell you your body is "attacking itself"? Do you constantly struggle with past events or current events you are unable to reconcile, which are a constant source of stress? These are all examples of catastrophizing thoughts, which are a heightened version of fear in which you project the worst possible outcomes in a never-ending negative loop in your mind. Catastrophizing can be defined as extremely negative thoughts and beliefs about pain.

Pain catastrophizing is a negative thought response to anticipated or actual pain and has been associated with poor physical function and negative outcomes in health and recovery. Catastrophizing is the inability to foresee anything other than the worst-case scenario, the tendency to describe a pain experience in more exaggerated terms than the average person or think an experience is unbearable when it's just uncomfortable, or to ruminate on it more frequently or obsessively. People who report a large number of such thoughts during a pain experience are more likely to rate the pain as more intense than those with fewer such thoughts.

PHYSICAL INJURY

Deconditioning
Depression
Diabesity

Avoidance

PAIN

Low
Fear   Confrontation   Healing
                                     & Recovery

Catastrophizing   Fear

**EMOTIONAL INJURY
& NEGATIVE THOUGHTS**

Constant feelings of fear, anger, and guilt are no fun and can keep you in a painful state. If most of your thoughts, feelings, and emotions are centered on your pain, your life can seem like one giant catastrophe. Pain-catastrophizing behaviors can influence the frequency and intensity of your pain. Here are some examples of pain-catastrophizing thoughts:

- *This pain is ruining my* entire *life.*
- *This pain is* killing *me.*
- *This is* never *going to get better.*

- *This is* only *going to get progressively worse.*
- *This pain interferes with* everything.

It is generally assumed that the tendency to catastrophize plays a role in the pain experience—that is, it may cause you to experience pain as more intense. Catastrophizing may influence pain perception by altering your attention and anticipation, and heightening emotional responses to pain. While catastrophizing thoughts have not yet been proven to always lead to more pain and suffering, all of the evidence indicates that catastrophizing about pain makes situations worse.

If you find yourself getting caught up in attack thoughts and catastrophizing, what can you do? You can make a conscious effort to change your thoughts and behaviors. Learn to get your body into the opposite state of the stress response, and change your script. Your brain is creating a movie, scripting whether you have pain. At times, illness or beliefs about illness have a strong hold over the mind and render you incapable of healing or believing in healing. The body can react inappropriately when responding to misthought, but only the mind is truly capable of error. The body cannot create pain, and the belief that it can, a fundamental error, produces all physical symptoms. Once you truly understand and accept the power of your thoughts, you can begin training your mind to conquer your pain (more on this in Chapter 10).

The Five Faces of Fears

The list of stressful or threatening thoughts and emotions you have on a daily basis can be significant, especially if you struggle with persistent pain. It should be well understood now that fear is a major obstacle in overcoming your pain and returning to an active life. Many things can cause fear, avoidance, and catastrophizing, but five themes typically surface in the clients I have worked with, and recognizing them will help you in your journey through the Healing Pain Program. The five fears include: failed treatment, financial issues, family stress, fear of movement, and fear of diagnosis. All of these fears are extremely powerful and not only lead you to avoid activity and catastrophize your situation but also cause serious stress, which signals danger in your brain.

The Five Fears

- Failed treatment
- Financial issues
- Family stress
- Fear of movement
- Fear of diagnosis

Failed Treatment

If you struggle with persistent pain, likely you have tried multiple ways to relieve your symptoms before and nothing has worked. You may have seen many doctors, therapists, and healers but still continue in your struggles. When you place your trust in one or multiple practitioners and do not receive results, it can be disappointing. In the end, you may be left feeling that treatment failed and you are doomed to live a life in pain and with decreased activity. Take note if you are feeling this way, because it may be affecting your ability to fully recover.

Financial Issues

On your quest for transformation, you may have discovered that the US health-care system is a sticky web that can be a financial trap. You may have started with your family care doctor only to be referred to a number of specialists in an effort to diagnose the problem correctly.

Top Five Financial Fears

- Mounting medical bills
- Missed work time
- Inability to perform financially
- Unemployment
- Disability

You may have also been taken through a battery of tests, including X-rays, MRIs, CT scans, blood work, stool samples, and so on. The maze of practitioners and tests can be expensive, with copayments, deductibles, and out-of-pocket expenses adding up significantly. If your health is poor, you may be out of work, working part-time, or missing work frequently.

Family Stress

This is perhaps one of the most challenging areas for my patients. Those who struggle with pain are often in the middle of their life. On one side, they may have children and a spouse whom they need to care for; and on the other, they may have ever-increasingly elderly parents who rely on them for emotional, financial, and physical help. Or you may be living with someone who does not know how to fully support you. This typically comes in the form of an overprotective partner who unknowingly keeps you dependent or one who is not able to provide the proper emotional support needed to recover. Either can deter your efforts and keep you stuck or unhealthy.

Common Family Stresses

- Arguments/disagreements
- Money
- Differences in child rearing
- Caregiving for child or parent

Fear of Movement

Persistent pain can lead you to fear even the most basic daily activity, and the thought of seeing a doctor of physical therapy who can help you with healthy movement may intensify your fear and therefore your pain. You want your pain to be resolved 100 percent before you begin to move again. Your fear of reinjury is palpable, and you feel it's simply better to remain on your couch with your feet up. You may believe that you need to rest instead of recognizing that moving or exercising is a clinically proven way to overcome persistent pain.

Fear of Diagnosis

You paid your $1,000 deductible for the MRI the doctor insisted you needed, and now you are in the MRI machine, with metal knocking all around you and magnetic energy painting a picture of your inner workings. The radiology tech can't tell you anything, so you must wait five days to get back in to see your doctor. Clinicians have the task not only to serve you with a diagnosis but also to explain what the diagnosis means, what your prognosis is, and various treatment options. Often physicians do not have adequate time to thoroughly explain what the tests mean or the courage to tell you that there is nothing observably wrong and you must make lifestyle changes to feel better. At times a diagnosis can sound alarming to a patient, inciting fear and catastrophizing emotions.

Language That Can Cause Fear

- Your disks are *degenerating*.
- The X-ray is *positive* for arthritis.
- You *have* fibromyalgia.
- It's "wear and tear."
- We need to run a battery of tests.
- The tests were inconclusive.
- You will have to learn to "manage" pain.
- This is "chronic."

The language you use and hear can affect your pain. Such words as *degenerating*, *chronic*, and *ruptured* can engender fear—although often they have nothing to do with your recovery and prognosis. Try not to assume the worst while you await your diagnosis—it won't help. Remain optimistic and remember that whatever the prognosis, you *can* overcome your pain.

Now that you have a better understanding of how your body heals and why your brain may be the real reason behind your pain—as well as how powerful your thoughts and emotions are when it comes to the phases of healing—you can hopefully move beyond some of your fears and begin to improve your health. If you find that you are struggling with catastrophic thoughts and overall fear and anxiety, skip ahead to Chapter 10 for some mind-training techniques to help you feel better.

Ten Myths About Healing Pain

Many of our thoughts have likely become ingrained over time, and the internal beliefs that we hold about pain can create another issue. These can be equally damaging to our recovery. Some of these myths we create ourselves, but some are influenced by the information we receive from family, friends, doctors, and more. It's important to dispel these myths to be able to move forward. Read each one carefully and really think about those that apply to you. If you believe any of these myths, they may be holding you back and hindering your recovery.

Myth One: If I struggle with persistent pain, it's because my injury hasn't healed properly.

Myth Two: The only way to resolve my pain is by taking medication.

Myth Three: Pain means I should rest and not move.

Myth Four: If your doctor can't find anything medically wrong with you, it must be "all in your head or you must be imagining it."

Myth Five: The worse my injury, the worse my pain will be.

Myth Six: Imaging studies will tell me the cause of my pain.

Myth Seven: Pain only occurs if there is a physical injury.

Myth Eight: There is nothing I can do to speed the healing process.

Myth Nine: Surgery or injections are the only way to solve my persistent pain.

Myth Ten: Persistent or chronic pain can't be healed.

Dr. Joe's Pain Relief Reminders

- There are three phases to healing: inflammation, repair, and remodeling. If your pain continues after three months, your brain may be keeping you in pain.
- Your body has no pain receptors; the brain decides on pain.
- Pain is both a sensory and emotional experience.
- Your emotions can influence your pain.
- Be aware of fear-avoidance behaviors and pain catastrophizing; they will hinder your recovery.
- The top five fears include: failed treatment, financial issues, family stress, fear of movement, and fear of diagnosis.

4

TEST, ASSESS, AND BEGIN

This chapter will take you on a journey, covering three essential areas that our traditional health-care system does not test. At the intersection of an active and healthy life free from pain and disability lies the assessment of your thoughts, movement, and nutrition—all of which are probably missing from your yearly physical. Your specific health decline may be related to one or all parts of this equation. But you must be able to assess where you are in each paradigm, because your own self-assessment is the beginning of your path back to health. This is your dashboard, your report card.

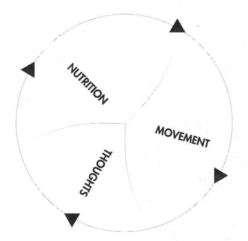

To help you with your self-assessment, this chapter offers a number of tests related to your current health, activity level, pain level, and perception as well as baseline measures of weight and overall wellness. Keep a record of your initial responses, so that you can measure your progress and transformation as you move through the Healing Pain Program. The tests may also enable you to determine which areas you are most deficient in and where you require the most assistance. For example, you may be doing well with your overall nutrition, but you need to work on your mind-set to become more comfortable with movement.

My Pain Story

You may think someone young and active would not encounter pain, but that's often not the case. Unfortunately, for me it developed right when I was in the middle of my university studies to become a physical therapist. Physical therapy is an incredibly demanding degree and requires many hours and years of study, learning about how the body and brain works. As a student you spend countless hours sitting in a chair. Classes ran most days from eight a.m. to six p.m. After lectures, I would escape for a quick dinner break and then return to the library for more studying. Most nights I would study until two a.m. For the first time in my life, I was sedentary for many hours and had a lot of stress, which was tough and depressing. Some days I would sit for more than fifteen hours! Intense back pain began to take me down. (You'll see later how sitting causes pain and weight gain, and I'll teach you how to prevent this.) I was twenty-four years old, a former gymnast, and a physical therapy student. I shouldn't have been in pain!

Luckily for me, I was around a team of accomplished physical therapy professors who treated me immediately, before it became chronic. I know you may have not been so lucky. However, I, too, fell prey to the trap of the medical system. My first step was to visit student health for an evaluation by a physician. My physician proceeded to order an MRI for me and prescribed a strong anti-inflammatory drug. Having already been halfway through my studies, I knew MRIs were not needed to effectively treat back pain. I refused and saved myself time and expense. I did, however, take the prescribed anti-inflammatories, which mildly helped the pain but had the awful side effect of ulcerlike symptoms.

My second experience with back pain was in 2010. This time I was educated and knew exactly what to do. The exercises I self-prescribed helped tremendously, but on some days, for reasons unbeknownst to me, the pain would creep back. This is when I really started to understand that back pain is not simply about the flexibility and strength of your spine. It's also about the many stressors we have in our life. At this time in my life, I had a busy practice, worked far too many hours, wasn't eating well, had financial pressures like rent and a mortgage, and was grieving the loss of a close family member. I was stressed, overworked, sleeping poorly, and didn't have enough time to dedicate to my own self-care. I was too busy taking care of everyone else—my patients and family came first. But that couldn't last forever. I realized that I had to work on the other two essential areas—nutrition and mind-set—and incorporate better eating habits and certain relaxation strategies into my life so as to feel better. The following questionnaire can help you evaluate your overall health and some of the areas that may be affecting your pain.

10-Step Recovery Questionnaire

Score 1 for yes and 0 for no.

1. Do you sleep fewer than seven hours each night? _____
2. Do you eat a diet of processed foods 50 percent of the time? _____
3. Do you exercise less than twice per week? _____
4. Do you currently struggle with depression or anxiety? _____
5. Have you had surgery to address a painful joint? _____
6. Do you have a history of physical or emotional abuse? _____
7. Would you rate your stress level as moderate to high? _____
8. Are you currently overweight? _____
9. Do you lack social support to help with your recovery? _____
10. Do you rely on pain medication to decrease your pain? _____

Total score _____

continues

10-Step Recovery Questionnaire *continued*

What Your Score Means

7 and above: The Healing Pain Program can help you with the strategies necessary for beginning the recovery process. You should make your health a priority and learn as much as you can about the lessons in the Healing Pain Diet, Movement, and Mind Programs.

4 to 6: Healing is needed to prevent further health problems. Use the Healing Pain Program as a guide to help you in areas that are lacking or where you need further education and inspiration.

1 to 3: Congratulations, you have a grasp on some of the essential habits to live a life free from persistent pain. With just a few more positive lifestyle changes, you will be on your way to living a healthy life and be a positive role model for friends and family.

Stress and Your Health

After reading Chapter 3, you should be well aware of the profound effects stress can have on your body—both mentally and physically. One of the first areas we will assess is stress, because it can have such a profound impact on your overall health. Your mind will personify your emotions, and they will inhabit far-reaching parts of your body. Stress can lead to muscle tension, tightness, and pain. And if you are under chronic stress, you will not be able to burn fat as easily as those who are not stressed.

Acquiring an understanding of how stress affects your health and developing an awareness around exactly how much stress you currently have in your life is a great place to begin. Your daily struggle with your health has repercussions in all areas of your life, and it's a two-way street. Identifying your overall level of stress and where the stressors live can be a solid beginning to your recovery. Take the following 10-Step Stress Questionnaire and see how you rate in terms of stress level. If your level is high, think about ways for reducing your stress (see Chapter 10 for some helpful tools). You can then take this test again after you've completed the Healing Pain Mind Program, to see whether your mood has improved.

10-Step Stress Questionnaire

Score 1 for yes and 0 for no.

1. Do you get fewer than seven hours of quality sleep each night? _____
2. Do you struggle financially or have you recently had a hardship? _____
3. Are you mourning the death of a friend or family member? _____
4. Have you recently been diagnosed with a disease or injury? _____
5. Do you exercise fewer than two days a week? _____
6. Do you lack a relaxation practice (meditation, prayer, etc.)? _____
7. Are you unhappy or dissatisfied at your current job? _____
8. Have you recently moved or relocated? _____
9. Have you been separated from a loved one or divorced? _____
10. Do you have thoughts of loneliness or lack love? _____

Total score _____

What Your Score Means

1 to 3: We all struggle with stress in our life. Fewer than three points on this quiz indicates that stress may not be an overwhelming factor in your life at this time.

4 to 10: Stress is a contributing factor to your pain. When stress becomes overwhelming or you lack buffering strategies, it can contribute to and sustain pain in your life. Learning a few techniques to buffer stress in your life will contribute to healing from your pain. For a more in-depth assessment of lifestyle contributors to pain, visit www .drjoetatta.com.

Are Negative Thoughts Inhibiting Recovery?

Catastrophic thinking literally affects the intensity of the pain you feel, leaving you in a constant state of stress. In many cases, catastrophic thoughts lead to increased pain and emotional distress, all increasing the probability that pain will persist over an extended period of time. If you can learn to minimize catastrophic thinking, you can reduce the persistence of your pain. The relationship between pain catastrophizing, fear, and depression is consistent. Pain catastrophizing might contribute to the development or persistence of anxiety, fear, or depression associated with pain.

Pain Catastrophizing Scale*

Everyone experiences painful situations at some point in their life. Such experiences may include headaches, tooth pain, joint pain, or muscle pain. People are often exposed to situations that may cause pain, such as illness, injury, procedures, or surgery.

     This test assesses the types of thoughts and feeling that you have when you are in pain. The following are thirteen statements describing different thoughts and feelings that may be associated with pain. Using the scale, please indicate the degree to which you have these thoughts and feelings when you are experiencing pain.

	Not at all	To a slight degree	To a moderate degree	To a great degree	All the time
I worry all the time about whether the pain will end.	0	1	2	3	4
I feel I can't go on.	0	1	2	3	4
It's terrible and I think it's never going to get any better.	0	1	2	3	4
It's awful and I feel that it overwhelms me.	0	1	2	3	4
I feel I can't stand it anymore.	0	1	2	3	4
I become afraid that the pain will get worse.	0	1	2	3	4
I keep thinking of other painful events.	0	1	2	3	4
I anxiously want the pain to go away.	0	1	2	3	4
I can't seem to keep it out of my mind.	0	1	2	3	4
I keep thinking about how much it hurts.	0	1	2	3	4
I keep thinking about how badly I want the pain to stop.	0	1	2	3	4
There's nothing I can do to reduce the intensity of the pain.	0	1	2	3	4
I wonder whether something serious may happen.	0	1	2	3	4

Total each column and then add them to calculate your score.

Total _____

A total score of greater than 30 represents a relevant level of catastrophizing.

*M. J. L. Sullivan, S. R. Bishop, and J. Pivik, "The Pain Catastrophizing Scale: Development and Validation," *Psychological Assessment* 7 (1995): 524–32.

Measure Your Body to Change Your Body

Once you have a handle on your mood and how stress can have an impact on your recovery, it's time for some basic physical body measurements or assessments, before we get into the specifics of nutrition and movement—both of which will affect your weight. I understand how challenging it can be to look at a number you don't want to see. But let me share one of the greatest weight-loss secrets with you: What gets measured gets improved! I want you to weigh yourself daily. This will provide you with the visual information necessary and act as the motivation and strength to avoid potential pitfalls on the weekend.

Be sure to record your numbers in a journal. In a 2015 study in the *Journal of Obesity*, 162 overweight individuals were placed into two groups—an intervention group or a delayed treatment control group. The members of the intervention group were given instructions to weigh themselves every morning and document their weight. Both groups received the same simple education on dietary strategies, such as skipping desserts, replacing a meal with a protein shake, and abstaining from snacks on most days. After one year, without any changes to diet or exercise, the participants receiving the intervention lost an average of 2 percent of their body weight and kept off the weight.

Several studies have included self-weighing as a component of behavioral weight loss. Keeping track of your numbers in a journal each day will keep you on track and provide you with feedback. Combined with the other strategies you will learn in the Healing Pain Diet Program, you will be on the road to recovery in no time.

Keep in mind that the number on a scale simply tells us the combined weight of all our tissue, including bone, muscle, and fat. As you will see in the later chapters, muscle is vitally important, although it weighs more than fat. If you are gaining muscle at the same time you are losing fat, you may not see the number on the scale drop as quickly as you would like. Remember, your weight is only one measurement; focus on the other outcomes in the Healing Pain Program, such as your pain, movement, nutrition, and thoughts. It is possible for the number on the scale to remain constant but still experience decreases in fat mass and increases in lean muscle mass.

Waist Circumference

While BMI may give an individual a general idea of increased risk for obesity-related health problems, the measurement of waist circumference provides insight into increased risk for obesity-related illness due to the *location* of excess fat. In fact, studies in both the *American Journal of Clinical Nutrition* and the *International Journal of Obesity* found a person's waist circumference is a better indicator of potential health problems than body mass index. You may have heard of fruit-based descriptions of body shape—apple shaped versus pear shaped. These fruits are used to describe the body fat distribution. Apple-shaped individuals carry the majority of their fat around the middle (abdominal fat), while the pears carry most of their fat around the hips (gluteal fat). If you have a "beer belly" but relatively thin legs, you're an apple. If you've ever been described as having an hourglass figure, you're a pear. Apples have a higher risk of disease and premature death than pears, so in terms of health, abdominal fat (apple) is worse for you than glute and hip fat (pear).

Part of why abdominal or belly fat is the worst kind of fat is because it includes both subcutaneous fat and visceral fat. Subcutaneous fat sits just under your skin, but visceral fat sits deep in your abdominal cavity and twists around your internal organs. In small amounts, visceral fat is good because it pads your organs, but in large amounts, visceral fat is a problem. Too much visceral fat has been linked to systemic inflammation—and we know that inflammation causes pain and more weight gain.

Waist circumference can be measured by placing a flexible cloth tape measure around the smallest part of the waist while standing relaxed. Waist circumference should be at or below 40 inches for men and 35 inches for women. Weight located in the trunk area places an individual at greater risk for high blood pressure, metabolic syndrome, type 2 diabetes, high cholesterol, coronary artery disease, and, of course, chronic pain syndromes! A larger waist circumference is correlated with almost every chronic, persistent pain syndrome, including osteoarthritis, rheumatoid arthritis and other autoimmune diseases, fibromyalgia, and disorders of pain sensitivity or hyperalgesia. For example, a 2015 study in the *European Journal of Pain* revealed a positive association between central body fat (waist or belly fat) and symptoms of pain and fatigue in 458 women with fibromyalgia.

Your waist circumference, or the length around your midsection, is a valuable piece of knowledge in determining your health risk due to excess body fat, and you can use it as a measure of your progress. While a waist circumference measurement is not a direct measurement of abdominal body fat percentage, keep track of this measurement as you improve with the Healing Pain Diet Program.

How to Measure Your Waist Circumference

Items you will need:

- Tape measure
- Partner or friend

Step 1: Stand upright and relaxed. Make sure your posture is straight up and down, with no bending or slouching. Let your arms hang loosely at your sides.

Step 2: Find the measurement site. You can find your true natural waist by following the horizontal line of your belly button. To make sure you have the correct spot, place your hands on your hips and bend sideways. The place where your waist indents or bends from is your natural waist.

Step 3: Measure with the tape measure. Have a partner do the actual measurement so that you can remain standing up straight. Have your partner place one end of the measuring tape right at your belly button and wind it around your waist until the tape measure comes back to overlap with the end. Do not cinch the tape measure tight, but simply let the tape rest on your skin for the measurement.

Step 4: Record the measurement. Keep track of your waist circumference over time to see changes.

Tip: For an accurate result, make sure the tape measure is completely horizontal during the measurement and not sagging down your back. It is best to perform this measurement with no clothing around the waist to prevent an overestimation of circumference measurement.

Nutrition: Is Your Diet Influencing Your Pain?

Who hasn't seen or heard Hippocrates's famous quote about letting food be your medicine and your medicine your food? This is an old concept coined by the Greek physician considered one of the most outstanding figures in the history of medicine. You may not yet understand how food can heal you, but you should understand that healthy nutrition is needed for weight loss and pain relief. Nutrition is a topic that could span a library full of books and require a PhD in biochemistry. However, the habits needed to live a nutritionally healthy life are simple. Quite frankly, we should teach this to our children from a very early age, engraining lasting habits that will permeate through our families and communities. The average American lacks any solid type of nutritional understanding, and most medical practitioners don't focus on this or educate their patients about it.

Musculoskeletal pain and inflammation can be caused by nutritional imbalances. Unfortunately, nutrition is an area where most medical professionals receive little training; providing nutritional advice would likely improve patient outcomes. According to a 2006 study in the *American Journal of Clinical Nutrition,* on average medical students received 23.9 contact hours of nutrition instruction during medical school. Medical school is a four-year process at minimum, so fewer than 25 hours of nutritional training reveals an alarming lack of emphasis on this critical area.

Nutrition is the fastest way to change your health, resolve your pain, and lose weight. This is your beginning. Answer the following questionnaire to assess your overall nutritional health and which areas may need work.

Movement: Assessing Your Activity Level

Movement is essential for a healthy life and is necessary to overcome pain. We will delve into more detail about the available options for healthy movement and exercise later in the book. In this section, I want you to have a baseline of where you are now, regarding how comfortable you feel around movement and where you may have deficits.

Nutrition Questionnaire

Score 1 for yes and 0 for no.

1. Do you eat a meal every four to six hours? _____

2. Does each meal include a source of lean protein? _____

3. Does each meal include at least three servings of vegetables? _____

4. Does each meal include 1 to 3 servings of healthy fat? _____

5. Does your dinner plate have a rainbow of colorful items? _____

6. Do you eat *only* one plate of food at each meal (no seconds)? _____

7. Do you limit starchy carbohydrate portions to less than a quarter of your plate? _____

8. Do you limit snacking? _____

9. Do you take a multivitamin and mineral supplement and omega-3 fish oil? _____

10. Have you eliminated gluten 100 percent from your diet? _____

Total score _____

What Your Score Means

4 to 10: Your habits when it comes to nutrition are in line with the guidelines of this program. Keep up the good work and try to get your score as close to 10 as possible.

0 to 3: If you answered no to more than three items or you were unsure, you will find helpful strategies in Chapters 5 through 7. Take this quiz again after you've completed the Healing Pain Diet Program and see whether you can answer yes to nearly all of the questions.

You should be able to move well right into your advanced years, enjoy a physically active life, and not have problems with basic activities of daily living. In our modern society, we have invented all types of machines to help us achieve tasks faster and more efficiently, but these often cause us to be more sedentary. However, we cannot forget about what we need to keep our own body healthy. In the following Pain and Movement Assessment, you can judge where your physical ability lies. After you have integrated the Healing Pain Movement Program into your life, reevaluate your movement to see how much you've improved.

Pain and Movement Assessment

Answer each question with never (0), seldom (1), sometimes (2), or often (3).

1. Pain prevents me from walking more than ¼ mile. _____

2. The pain prevents me from playing with my kids or grandkids. _____

3. The pain prevents me from sitting for more than an hour. _____

4. The pain prevents me from exercising, the gym, or fitness. _____

5. The pain interferes with my ability to sleep. _____

6. The pain interferes with my ability to bend and lift objects from the floor. _____

7. The pain prevents me from participating in social activities with friends. _____

8. The pain prevents me from standing for more than 30 minutes. _____

9. During conversation, I zone out and can't concentrate due to pain. _____

10. I have to rely on pain relief pills to live my daily life. _____

11. When I am under stress, my pain increases. _____

12. The pain interferes with my ability to do household chores. _____

13. The pain has caused me to gain weight due to inactivity. _____

14. I have noticed a correlation with my weight and the frequency of my pain. _____

15. I've had chronic pain for years, and it hasn't improved. _____

Total score _____

What Your Score Means

21 and above: Your struggle is affecting your quality of life. You need to incorporate the strategies in the Healing Pain Movement Program to help alleviate your pain now and lose weight.

10 to 20: You display some symptoms of persistent pain and would benefit from the Healing Pain Movement Program to reduce your pain and weight.

Below 10: While you suffer little to no symptoms, adopting a few new strategies from the Healing Pain Movement Program will maximize your health and vitality.

Systemic Inflammatory Symptoms

Chronic inflammation from lifestyle choices can have far-reaching effects on the body. You likely have aches and pains in muscles and joints and your weight has been a challenge. It is also important for you to be able to make the connection on how inflammation is affecting areas and systems of your body. Everything in your body is interwoven in a web. When one system is off, it will have a significant impact on other parts of the body.

After taking the following quiz, you may realize you have problems that center on your joints, skin, and digestion, or you have problems with energy and weight. Many of your symptoms are connected, and beginning the Healing Pain Program will be your path to alleviating them. Most clients find that once they incorporate the strategies into their life, they begin not only to see their weight and pain decrease but also are pleased with the added benefit of having increased energy, improved mood, less digestive problems, better skin, and a host of other positive physical and mental improvements. Take the quiz now and retake it once you have completed four weeks on the program.

How Bad Is Your Inflammation?

Use the following inflammation index to rate each of the following symptoms based upon your typical health profile for the past thirty days. In addition to contributing to pain, inflammation can affect many body systems and organs. Use the following scale to rate yourself from 0 (no symptoms) to 3 (severe symptoms).

Point Scale

0: Never have symptoms
1: Minimal symptoms

2: Moderate symptoms
3: Severe symptoms

HEAD

_____ Headaches or migraines
_____ Dizziness
_____ Trouble sleeping
_____ Faintness
_____ **TOTAL**

EYES

_____ Watery or itchy eyes
_____ Red or swollen eyelids
_____ Bags or dark circles under eyes
_____ Vision problems
_____ **TOTAL**

continues

How Bad Is Your Inflammation? *continued*

EARS

_____ Itchy ears
_____ Earaches
_____ Drainage from ear
_____ Ringing or hearing loss
_____ **TOTAL**

NOSE

_____ Stuffy nose
_____ Sinus problems
_____ Hay fever
_____ Sneezing attacks
_____ Excessive mucus formation
_____ **TOTAL**

THROAT

_____ Chronic coughing
_____ Frequent need to clear throat
_____ Sore throat or hoarseness
_____ Discolored tongue, gums, lips
_____ **TOTAL**

SKIN

_____ Acne
_____ Rash or hives
_____ Hair loss
_____ Hot flashes
_____ Excessive sweating
_____ **TOTAL**

HEART

_____ Irregular heartbeat
_____ Racing or pounding heartbeat
_____ Chest pain
_____ **TOTAL**

LUNGS

_____ Chest congestion
_____ Asthma, bronchitis
_____ Shortness of breath
_____ Difficulty breathing
_____ **TOTAL**

DIGESTION

_____ Nausea, vomiting
_____ Diarrhea
_____ Constipation
_____ Bloating
_____ Gas
_____ Heartburn
_____ Stomach pain
_____ **TOTAL**

MUSCULOSKELETAL

_____ Pain or aches in joints
_____ Arthritis
_____ Stiffness or limitation of movement
_____ Pain in muscles
_____ Feeling of weakness
_____ **TOTAL**

WEIGHT

_____ Excessive weight
_____ Binge eating
_____ Cravings
_____ Compulsive eating
_____ **TOTAL**

continues

How Bad Is Your Inflammation? *continued*

ENERGY

_____ Fatigue, sluggishness
_____ Lethargic
_____ Hyperactivity
_____ Restlessness
_____ **TOTAL**

MOOD

_____ Mood swings
_____ Anxiety, fear, nervousness
_____ Anger, irritability
_____ Depression
_____ **TOTAL**

BRAIN

_____ Poor memory
_____ Confusion
_____ Brain fog
_____ Difficulty making decisions
_____ Speech problems
_____ **TOTAL**

_____ **GRAND TOTAL**

Add up your totals and notice the specific areas where you seem to have the most issues. After completing the Healing Pain Program, take the quiz again and see whether your total score has decreased and/or some of your problem areas have improved. Many who struggle with persistent pain often have higher symptoms in the categories of musculoskeletal, digestion, mood, and brain.

Hopefully, this chapter enabled you to perform some tests of your own to better determine your current health status when it comes to thoughts, movement, and nutrition and to identify the problem areas that especially need work. Having a baseline assessment helps you truly see where you are now and compare that to how you feel after you complete the Healing Pain Program.

Dr. Joe's Pain Relief Reminders

- What gets measured gets improved.
- Take each test before starting the Healing Pain Program.
- Retake each test at the end of three weeks to measure your progress.

Part II

The Healing Pain Diet Program

5

CORE NUTRITIONAL HEALING

The Basics of Core Nutritional Healing

Goal: Strive to make all the changes in this phase immediately. These are foundational principles of nutrition to be followed for a healthy and pain-free life.

Changes: Eliminate highly processed foods, food additives, trans fats, and toxins that contribute to pain and disease, adding in healthful whole foods high in phytonutrients, vitamins, minerals, antioxidants, fiber, and healthy fats.

Results: Moderate decrease in pain down 2 pain points, average weight loss of 5 to 7 pounds within two weeks.

Nutrition is your foundation for healing from pain and losing weight, and food is the medicine that will deliver it to you. Bad food is bad medicine and will harm your health. Good food is good medicine and can prevent—and even cure—disease. Eliminate the bad food, replace it with the good food, and magical healing occurs. This approach is better than any medication and provides concrete, sustained results. The power of this simple diet change—getting rid of the harmful foods and consuming the healthful foods—can often reverse the most difficult-to-treat chronic diseases and give people the experience of profound wellness.

Many chronic health problems, such as pain and obesity, are the result of measurable imbalances in the body's biochemistry that can be corrected with proper nutrition. They are typically caused by various long-term combinations of stress, poor diet, lack of exercise, inflammation, insulin resistance, infections, and/or toxic exposures (whose effects can persist in the body for decades), as well as genetic differences. Despite the fact that many of the lifestyle factors are modifiable, most of the treatments you have received come in the form of a pill or procedure, such as an injection, painkiller, or surgery.

In this chapter you will discover just how powerful the right nourishment can be for healing, and you will see how what you choose to eat can have a strong impact on your health, pain relief, and weight. Let's think of core nutritional healing as Nutrition 101. I'll explain which of your current habits may be damaging your health, where you may have important deficiencies, and what you *should* be incorporating into your diet and why, as you begin your nutritional transformation.

The SAD Beginning of Your Weight and Pain Struggles

How does your day begin? If you are like most Americans, you wake up feeling fatigued, bloated, and in pain. After being jolted out of bed by an alarm, you realize your first steps may be the most pain you are in all day. The plantar fascia on the bottom of your feet is screaming because it's so inflamed, your knees feel as stiff as the Tin Man in *The Wizard of Oz,* and your spine feels like an inflexible steel pole. Undoubtedly, some of your problems have to do with your sedentary life, but the standard American diet (SAD) you have been sustaining yourself on is, in fact, sustaining the chronic inflammation, pain, and extra weight. Stumbling into the kitchen, you reach for a mug of coffee and a waffle, or maybe you pick up an oversize latte and a bagel or doughnut at the drive-through. Your day—and your inflammation—is beginning.

The standard American diet is known to be proinflammatory, due to the overconsumption of simple, highly fermentable carbohydrates, food additives, trans-fatty acids, and vegetable oils as well as to dietary monotony. The SAD also provides less than optimal servings of fruits and vegetables, along with highly processed, high-caloric foods that are nutrient deficient. This dietary combination lacks fiber, phytonutrients, vitamins, minerals, and healthy fatty acids. Health-promoting fatty acids and phytonutrients are known to be anti-inflammatory in nature and can help you with your resistant weight loss and pain. Let's look at some of the most detrimental aspects of the SAD and its effect on your health.

A Lack of Healthy Fats

We have a plethora of research and information on how our current diet causes us to be painfully heavy, and one of the primary problems is a lack of healthy fats. Both omega-6 and omega-3 fatty acids are required by the body; however, an overabundance of omega-6 fatty acids are known to create a proinflammatory environment. While we do not have research studies on our ancestors going back thousands of years, we do know some things about their diet. In prehistoric times, the ratio of omega-6 fatty acids (linoleic, arachidonic acid) to omega-3 fatty acids (alpha-linolenic acid, eicosapentaenoic acid, docosahexaenoic acid) was close to 1:1. Our ancestors consumed foods obtained from hunting and foraging, and their omega-3 fatty acid intake (found in fish and free-range meat) was 5,000 to 10,000 milligrams per day. The current SAD can cause fatty acid imbalances, because it is abundant in omega-6 fats (found in vegetable oils, corn oil, margarine, and processed foods), which promote inflammation. The Healing Pain Diet Program will improve your fatty acid balance and help restore your health. Omega-3 fatty acid deficiencies further contribute to an inflammatory cascade. A proinflammatory diet can excite the nociceptors that signal pain.

Our omega-6 to omega-3 ratio must be less than 4:1 to avoid inflammatory chronic diseases. With the SAD, fatty acid imbalances exist in the range of 15:1. Studies have demonstrated that Inuit who eat a traditional diet high in omega-3 fatty acids and low in omega-6 acids are almost free of chronic degenerative diseases commonly found in Western cultures, supporting evidence that omega-3 fatty acids exert an anti-inflammatory effect.

> ## Our Lean and Pain-Free Ancestors
>
> No traditional group followed a vegetarian diet.
> None was a low-fat diet.
> Food was local, natural, and whole.
> All had some raw or probiotic foods.
> All were unprocessed, organic, and free of chemicals.

Treacherous Trans Fats

In addition to lacking in healthy fats, the standard American diet contains far too many unhealthy trans fats. Trans fats, often labeled "partially hydrogenated," are not found anywhere in nature. Our ancestral diet didn't include them and I avoid them like the plague—and so should you! They exist in processed foods, such as cookies, crackers, and cakes. Any vegetable oil (soybean, corn, canola, safflower, sunflower, and so on) can be either partially hydrogenated or nonhydrogenated (the latter do not contain trans fats). Some experts will tell you that you can have up to 2 grams of trans fats per day. I say, *No way.* There is no place for trans fats in your diet.

Trans fats can double your risk of heart disease by raising your LDL (bad cholesterol) and lowering your HDL (good cholesterol). The inflammatory trans-fat pathway leads to inflammation of the blood vessels, coronary heart disease, and increased mortality. And clogged arteries can affect more than your heart. Atherosclerosis can block leg arteries, causing a condition known as vascular claudication. Vascular claudication produces a cramping pain in the buttocks, thighs, or calves caused by impaired blood flow to the legs, which can make walking difficult. Studies have revealed an association between atherosclerosis in the aorta and degenerative disk disease, as well as between blocked arteries in the lower back and lifetime low back pain.

Too Many Processed Foods

You also likely consume far too many processed foods. Most of these foods can be found in the center aisles of your supermarket and they come in the form of a box, can, or bottle, with a long list of unidentifiable ingredients. They include such items as soda, cookies, cake mixes, potato chips, and meals that can be made from a packet or heated up quickly in a microwave. A recent study from the University of North Carolina at Chapel Hill found that most Americans obtain 60 percent of their calories from highly processed foods. No wonder why so many Americans are in pain and overweight! In addition to large quantities of sugar and unhealthy omega-6 fats, processed foods also often contain dangerous substances, such as food additives, preservatives, and artificial sweeteners.

Food Additives: Tasty but Deadly

Food additives are a one-way ticket to pain and may even lead to weight gain. The two most widely used food additives are MSG (monosodium glutamate) and aspartate, both of which are known as excitotoxins. Excitotoxins are molecules that act as excitatory neurotransmitters and can lead to neurotoxicity. Neurotoxicity leads to cell death, and when cells die, inflammation and pain is sure to follow. Aspartate and glutamate act as neurotransmitters in the brain by facilitating the transmission of information from neuron to neuron. Too much aspartate or glutamate in the brain kills certain neurons by allowing the influx of too much calcium into the cells. This influx triggers excessive amounts of free radicals, which kill the cells. They "excite," or stimulate, the neurons and entice them to early cellular death.

Most people are familiar with MSG as a flavor enhancer used in Chinese food. What you may not realize is that it's also found in many processed foods. In studies, MSG seems to have the same impact on chronic pain conditions as artificial sweeteners. Glutamate, a component of MSG, can damage nerve endings when taken in excess. When this occurs, there is an amplification of pain. Today, MSG is added to most convenience foods, soups, chips, frozen foods, ready-made dinners, and canned goods. It has been a blessing for the diet food industry, because so many of the low-fat foods are tasteless. Companies use MSG to bring the flavor of food alive, all while damaging your nervous system. Often MSG and related toxins added to foods are completely disguised by names that seem harmless. (See the following charts, which reveal the many different terms for MSG.)

In a study in the *Annals of Pharmacotherapy*, patients diagnosed with fibromyalgia syndrome for upward of seventeen years had complete, or nearly complete, resolution of their symptoms within months after eliminating MSG or MSG plus aspartame from their diet. All patients were women with multiple comorbidities prior to elimination of MSG. All have had recurrence of symptoms whenever MSG was reintroduced into their diet.

Hidden Sources of Processed Free Glutamic Acid (MSG)

These ALWAYS contain MSG		
Glutamate	Glutamic acid	Gelatin
Monosodium glutamate	Calcium caseinate	Textured protein
Monopotassium glutamate	Sodium caseinate	Yeast nutrient
Yeast extract	Yeast food	Autolyzed yeast
Hydrolyzed protein (any protein that is hydrolyzed)	Hydrolyzed corn gluten	Natrium glutamate (*natrium* is Latin/German for "sodium")

These OFTEN contain MSG or create MSG during processing:		
Carrageenan	Maltodextrin	Malt extract
Natural pork flavoring	Citric acid	Malt flavoring
Bouillon and broth	Natural chicken flavoring	Soy protein isolate
Natural beef flavoring	Ultrapasteurized	Soy sauce
Stock	Barley malt	Soy sauce extract
Whey protein concentrate	Pectin	Soy protein
Whey protein	Protease	Soy protein concentrate
Whey protein isolate	Protease enzymes	Anything protein fortified
Flavors(s) and flavoring(s)	Anything enzyme modified	Anything fermented
Natural flavor(s) and flavoring(s)	Anything enzymes	Seasonings (the word *seasonings*)

Painful Preservatives

One of the reasons that many foods can last so long on store shelves is due to the addition of preservatives—chemicals called by such names as benzoates, monoglycerides, diglycerides, nitrates, nitrites, and sulfites—that keep the food from spoiling. They are often found in commercially prepared baked goods, such as cookies or crackers. A number of studies have linked some of these preservatives to chronic pain conditions.

Achy Artificial Sweeteners

The negative impact of consuming sugar-sweetened beverages on weight and other health outcomes has been increasingly recognized, and we are learning there is no difference between table sugar and artificial sweeteners. Artificial sweeteners, such as sucralose and aspartame and their various trademarked names and chemical cousins, have no place in the Healing Pain Program. Some of the more common names for these sweeteners include NutraSweet, Equal, and Sweet'N Low—see the box on page 74 for an extensive list. Although most of these claim to be low-calorie or zero-calorie sweeteners, this can be deceiving. One study of 3,682 individuals examined the long-term relationship between consuming artificially sweetened drinks and weight. The participants were followed for seven to eight years and their weights were monitored. After adjusting for common factors that contribute to weight gain, such as dieting, a change in exercise habits, or diabetes status, the study revealed that those who drank artificially sweetened drinks had a 47 percent higher increase in BMI than did those who did not drink sweetened beverages.

One concern about artificial sweeteners is that they affect the body's ability to gauge how many calories are being consumed. Some studies show that sugar and artificial sweeteners affect the brain in different ways. Anything sweet sends a signal to the brain to eat more. By providing a sweet taste without any calories, artificial sweeteners cause us to crave more sweet foods and drinks, which can ultimately add up to excess calories. Just because something says it has zero calories does not mean it is harmless; it can still sabotage weight-loss efforts and even cause weight gain.

Many artificial sweeteners that contain aspartame, and Splenda, which contains sucralose, are found in diet drinks and foods as well as the little packets on restaurant tables. Evidence suggests that frequent consumers of these sugar substitutes may also be at increased risk of excessive weight gain, metabolic syndrome, type 2 diabetes, and cardiovascular disease.

Artificial sweetener	Brand names	Sweetness as compared to sugar
Aspartame	Equal, NutraSweet, others	180 times sweeter than sugar
Acesulfame-K	Sunett, Sweet One	200 times sweeter than sugar
Saccharin	Sweet'N Low, Necta Sweet, others	300 times sweeter than sugar
Sucralose	Splenda	600 times sweeter than sugar
Neotame	No brand names	7,000 times sweeter than sugar

Artificial sweeteners were developed as safe, healthy substitutes for sugar, but research has also linked these food additives to a variety of chronic pain conditions, including fibromyalgia and migraines. One of my patients who came in for chronic headaches drank three diet sodas every day and had been placed on two different types of pain medications for headache after an MRI, CT scan, and EEG of his brain. Once I removed the diet soda from his diet, his headaches disappeared. He also lost 5 pounds the first week, presumably from decreased cravings associated with artificial sweeteners, and was able to stop taking handfuls of Advil. The painful reality is that these artificial sweeteners are even more dangerous than actual sugar when it comes to losing weight and decreasing pain. If you need to use a sweetener, I recommend organic stevia, a plant native to South America. The plant's leaves are two hundred times sweeter than sugar; a little goes a long way. The advantages of stevia are it contains no carbohydrates or calories and won't raise blood sugar levels.

Overconsumption of Carbohydrates = High Blood Sugar and Insulin Resistance

Regulating blood sugar and insulin is vital in your attempts to lose weight, reduce pain, and reverse chronic inflammation. Certain foods have more of an impact on your blood sugar's spiking than others. Whereas fat and protein have little effect on blood sugar, carbohydrates directly affect its release. Insulin resistance often accompanies the most common complaints the Healing Pain Diet Program addresses—pain and weight gain. More than 80 million Americans suffer from insulin resistance, and it appears to sit at the center of a web of related health problems. If you are insulin resistant, you are at much greater risk for painful syndromes, obesity, diabetes, hypertension (high blood pressure), heart disease, and high cholesterol. There is even good evidence that insulin resistance may be implicated in Alzheimer's disease. With its highly processed, starchy, and sugary foods, the standard American diet increases blood sugar, which then leads to insulin resistance.

Insulin is a hormone that facilitates the transport of sugar (glucose) from the bloodstream into cells throughout the body for use as fuel. In response to the normal increase in blood sugar after a meal, the pancreas secretes insulin into the bloodstream. With insulin resistance, the normal amount of insulin secreted is not sufficient to move glucose into the cells, or due to the high and constant blood sugar levels, it is toxic to your cells and stops the uptake of glucose—thus the cells are said to be "resistant." To compensate, the pancreas secretes insulin in ever-increasing amounts to maintain fairly adequate blood-sugar movement into cells and a normal blood-sugar level. The goal is to keep your blood sugar stable and avoid large spikes that cause an increase in insulin, which will rapidly convert carbohydrates into fat and cause chronic inflammation and pain. Understanding carbohydrates and how they affect your body can be a challenge but also a key to maximizing your weight loss. Diet and exercise can improve insulin sensitivity, lowering chronic inflammation, pain, and weight gain.

Understanding both the glycemic index and the glycemic load can blaze a path for fast fat loss. The glycemic index (GI) is a numerical system of measuring how much of a rise in blood sugar a carbohydrate triggers—the higher the number, the greater the blood sugar response. So, a low-GI food will cause a small rise, whereas a high-GI food will trigger a dramatic spike in blood sugar. A GI of 70 or more is high, a GI of 56 to 69 is medium, and a GI of 55 or less is low.

The glycemic load (GL) is a relatively new way to assess the impact of carbohydrate consumption that takes the glycemic index into account while giving a fuller picture than the GI alone. A GI value tells you only how rapidly a particular carbohydrate turns into sugar. It doesn't tell you how much of that carbohydrate is in a serving of a particular food. You need to know both measurements to understand a food's effect on blood sugar. The carbohydrate in watermelon, for example, has a high GI. But there isn't a lot of it, so watermelon's glycemic load is relatively low. A GL of 20 or more is high, a GL of 11 to 19 is medium, and a GL of 10 or less is low. Don't feel like doing the math? Refer to the Healing Pain Diet food shopping list on pages 96–97. I have done the work for you. Now that you understand how carbohydrates can adversely affect your pain and weight loss, all you have to do is take the list to the grocery store with you and purchase foods from the list.

Picking the Perfect Fruit

Fruit can be deceiving and often be a ticket to feed your sweet tooth. The following guide will help you with your choices.

Low-glycemic fruit choices (pick these!): Apples, blackberries, blueberries, cherries, lemons, limes, pomegranates, raspberries, strawberries

Moderate-glycemic fruit choices (eat in moderation): Apricots, grapefruit, kiwis, melons, nectarines, oranges, passion fruit, peaches, pears, persimmons, plums, tangerines

High-glycemic fruit choices (avoid until you reach weight-loss goal!): Bananas, grapes, mangoes, papayas, pineapple, watermelon

An Abundance of Nutrient Deficiencies

The standard American diet causes numerous nutrient deficiencies. A 2010 study performed by the Institute of Medicine and published in the *Journal of Nutrition* concluded, "Nearly the entire U.S. population consumes a diet that is not on par with dietary recommendations." These findings have obvious implications for national health and chronic disease. Poor nutrition can cause deficiencies, and these deficiencies have a direct effect on your musculoskeletal pain.

Insufficient vitamin D is widespread in modern society, with reports of 40 to 80 percent of adult Americans suffering from a deficiency. Vitamin D is immune modulating, and a deficiency contributes to a proinflammatory state in the body and can cause musculoskeletal pain because it inhibits calcium absorption into the bones. Several studies have revealed that vitamin D deficiency is common in people with musculoskeletal pain and that correcting the deficiency can alleviate pain. Studies demonstrate that inadequate levels of vitamin D are found in those with chronic low back pain and alleviated when they took a vitamin D supplement. Vitamin D_3 is the most bioavailable for the human body and is quickly absorbed. Unfortunately, vitamin D is rarely found in any foods, so increasing your intake requires a supplement or time spent in the sun. Exposing your arms or legs to twenty to thirty minutes of indirect sunlight daily can provide you with all the vitamin D needed for a healthy life.

The B vitamin family is important for your nerve health and myelin sheath formation. The *Merck Manual* recommends 50 milligrams twice daily as a trial. Vitamins B_2 (riboflavin) and B_6 (pyridoxine) have been shown to alleviate carpel tunnel syndrome, and vitamin B_3 (niacin) has helped patients suffering with osteoarthritis. A recent study found that vitamin B_3 improved joint mobility, decreased inflammation, reduced the impact of arthritis on activities of daily living, and allowed a reduction of anti-inflammatory medication as compared to a placebo in seventy-two patients with osteoarthritis. The different types of vitamin B can be found in meat, fish, dairy, spinach, almonds, peanuts, mushrooms, avocados, beans, and eggs.

Vitamin E, with its antioxidant, anti-inflammatory, and analgesic effects, has long been used to treat musculoskeletal pain. In studies, 40 to 600 milligrams of vitamin E were used to treat patients with rheumatoid arthritis, with some reports of symptom relief, although further research is needed on dosage and efficacy. You can find vitamin E in sunflower seeds, almonds, spinach, red peppers, asparagus, fish, mangoes, and avocados.

Magnesium is required for hundreds of biochemical reactions and is one of the most abundant minerals in the body, yet studies report that 20 to 40 percent of people are magnesium deficient. A large US national survey indicated that the average magnesium intake is below the current recommended dietary allowance by about 350 milligrams per day for men and about 260 milligrams per day for women. Magnesium intakes were even lower in men and women over fifty years of age. There's a good chance that you aren't consuming adequate amounts of magnesium. Magnesium plays a key role in producing energy in muscle cells, so intake is critical during physical therapy, considering exercise is a primary form of treatment. Magnesium supplementation has been used to treat migraine headaches, as a deficiency is common in headache patients. Magnesium may also be beneficial for fibromyalgia patients, due to impaired mitochondria function. You can get more magnesium into your diet by consuming dark leafy greens, nuts, seeds, fish, beans, whole grains, avocados, and bananas.

In addition to vitamins and minerals, many people need more amino acids in their body. Amino acids are the building blocks of protein, and they make up the second largest component of muscles, cells, and tissues. They are also one of the major elements of neurotransmitters used for neuroendocrine communication. Patients recovering from an injury, surgery, or desiring muscle growth should receive proper amino acid intake. Amino acids have been used to alleviate pain and promote analgesia, and according to a recent study they can also improve symptoms from fibromyalgia. Adults should consume 50 to 300 milligrams per day. Foods with the highest sources of amino acids include lean meat, poultry, seafood, eggs, chia seeds, sunflower seeds, almonds, avocados, figs, and quinoa.

Finally, as we've already discussed, most of us don't receive adequate omega-3 fatty acids. The omega-3 fatty acids EPA and DHA generally occur together and have been used as a supplement to treat musculoskeletal and autoimmune conditions. Omega-3 fatty acids have anti-inflammatory properties and increase central serotonergic activity, which alleviates pain. They also stimulate the development of cartilage for joint repair and increase mineral absorption in your gut. Omega-3 fatty acid supplementation in clinical trials has been effective for migraine, low back pain, rheumatoid arthritis, and joint pain. Recommended supplemental dosages for treatment of musculoskeletal problems are approximately 3,000 milligrams of EPA and DHA. For more omega-3 fatty acids in your diet, be sure to consume walnuts, halibut, salmon, sardines, eggs, and cauliflower. You can refer to Appendix B (p. 305) for more recommendations on supportive supplements specific to your condition.

Medications Deplete Important Nutrients

Medications are not a food group, although by the way the average person consumes them you would think they are. Nearly 70 percent of Americans are on at least one prescription drug, and more than half receive at least two prescriptions. This does not account for over-the-counter medications, which are readily available and many of which are equally dangerous despite their availability without a prescription. No doubt that if you are overweight and struggle with pain, you are currently taking or have taken one or more types of medication to manage your symptoms.

Many people are on medication for years, without thinking twice about the ramifications. However, an underlying consequence of chronic medication use needs to be articulated. Nutrient depletions are common with medications and have widespread effects throughout the body. Certain medications and classes of medications can deplete your body and cells of certain nutrients and, in turn, cause pain. Nutrient depletions can have profound effects on your immune, musculoskeletal, digestive, endocrine, and neurological systems. Here are a few examples:

- **NSAIDs:** These include over-the-counter drugs, such as Advil, Aleve, and Excedrin. They can deplete iron, which can cause anemia and weaken

continues

Medications Deplete Important Nutrients *continued*

your immune system, vitamin B_9 (folic acid), vitamin C, and zinc, which can lead to a weakened immune system and increased susceptibility to infection.

- **Glucocorticoids:** These include such steroids as prednisone and cortisone. They can deplete magnesium, potassium, sodium, selenium, and zinc—all important minerals for bone health, cellular health, muscle and nerve function, and immune health. They can also reduce calcium absorption and may interfere with calcium and vitamin D metabolism.
- **DMARDs:** These include such medications as methotrexate, leflunomide, hydroxychloroquine, sulfasalazine, minocycline, azathioprine, and cyclosporine. Possible nutrient depletion includes vitamins B_3, B_6, B_9, and B_{12} (cyanocobalamin), and K; calcium, copper, iron, and magnesium; antioxidants, such as glutathione; and probiotics, such as lactobacillus.
- **Opioids:** These include drugs such as codeine, hydrocodone, Vicodin, oxycodone, and morphine. Common nutrient depletions are selenium, zinc, and glutathione.

Healing Pain Nutrient Protocols

Between the standard American diet and the impact from various medications, you will need a little help filling in some of your nutritional deficiencies to decrease inflammation, aid in rebuilding tissue, and assist in healing. And if you are like most of my patients, you are looking for not only relief of your pain in the fastest way possible but also the *safest* way possible. Supplementing your diet with some essential nutrients will work to complete your healing. I have included a cheat sheet here for you regarding the most important nutrients you should be taking. You will also find more healing pain nutrient protocols as you progress throughout this book, including important ones in the next chapter on gut healing. A comprehensive table is also available for you in Appendix B.

For Everyone		
Supplement	**Dosage**	**Notes**
Multivitamin/mineral	2x/day	Twice daily multivitamin and mineral
Omega-3 fatty acids EPA and DHA	3,000–5,000 mg/daily	Used to decrease inflammation, modulate pain, regulate blood sugar and cholesterol levels
Vitamin D_3	2,000 IU daily	Deficiencies of less than 50 ng/mL of vitamin D have been associated with inflammation, leaky gut, decreased healing, autoimmunity, migraines, and musculoskeletal pain.

Inflammation/Immune Support		
Supplement	**Dosage**	**Notes**
Curcumin	500 mg 2x/day	Contain natural plant-based antioxidant, anti-inflammatory, and immune stimulating properties to decrease inflammation. Positive effects have been noted with decreased reactive oxygen species, NF-kB, leukotriene, and prostaglandins, blood sugar, and fatty acid rebalancing.
Resveratrol	500 mg 2x/day	
N-acetyl-D-glucosamine	500 mg daily	
Ginger	200 mg 2x/day	
Skullcap	100 mg daily	
Proteolitic enzymes	200 mg 2x/day	
Boswellia	200 mg 2x/day	
Andrographis paniculata	2,000 mg 2x/day	

Joint Healing		
Supplement	**Dosage**	**Notes**
Glucosamine sulfate	1,000 mg daily	All are important nutrients and precursors for healthy joint tissue, structure, and function and found in cartilage, ligaments, tendons, and connective tissue.
Chondroitin sulfate	1,000 mg daily	
MSM (methulsulfonylmethane)	250 mg daily	
Collagen peptides	7 g daily	
Hyaluronic acid	40 mg daily	

continues

continued

Tension/Tightness		
Supplement	**Dosage**	**Notes**
Valerian root	200 mg 2x/day	Extracts of valerian and other
Passionflower	200 mg 2x/day	plant-based extracts may
Lemon balm	100 mg 2x/day	help reduce muscle pain and muscle tension through inducing relaxation, reducing anxiety, and
Magnesium	500 mg 2x/day	possibly mild sedation of the nervous system.

Muscle/Tissue Repair		
Supplement	**Dosage**	**Notes**
Branched-chain amino acids (BCAA) (leucine, isoleucine, valine, plus L-glutamine)	5–10 g	Branched-chain amino acids, along with L-glutamine, stimulate muscle synthesis even in the absence of resistance training, making them essential in those who are unable to exercise but are at risk for muscle loss (sarcopenia). BCAAs are also essential in sports nutrition— enhancing muscle building and recovery in athletes. BCAAs can also prevent sarcopenia postoperatively or after a traumatic injury, and muscle catabolism associated with inflammatory diseases.

The Five Steps to Start Core Healing

Now that you better understand why it's so important to avoid the overly processed standard American diet, consume healthy omega-3 fats, overcome vitamin and mineral deficiencies, and keep your blood sugar in check, we're going to focus on what you *should* be doing to begin healing your body from the inside out. This will include both eliminating the most problematic processed foods, as well as incorporating healing whole foods into your diet for the next few weeks. In this first phase of core nutritional healing, the aim is to fill your body with foods that are rich in antioxidants and phytonutrients as well as healthy fats, protein, and plenty of fiber.

#1 Eliminate Processed Foods

If you are intent on healing, it needs to begin with real, whole foods. Much of what you consume on a daily basis from breakfast to dinner and for snacks is as far from real food as you can get. The Healing Pain Diet Program is your reintroduction to what real whole food actually *is* and why you should stay as far away as possible from all other sources. Real whole foods are those that are grown in a natural life cycle rather than manufactured in a laboratory or factory. These are also foods that have nothing added or removed between when they are picked and when they are purchased. Knowing this is the safest way to ensure that the nutrients naturally found in the food are intact and no additives—such as synthetic preservatives or artificial colorings or flavorings, artificial sweeteners, hormones, or antibiotics—have been added. You should begin eliminating these harmful substances from your diet.

Food marketing has twisted our thinking as to what is actually food. Breads, pizza, pasta, and pies or processed meats, such as chicken tenders, are not whole foods. It may seem challenging at first to remove these processed foods from your meals, but if you want to heal your pain, it starts with what you choose to put into your body. Want to make your food taste better? It's incredible what a pinch of sea salt, dried oregano, or fresh thyme can do. Herbs and spices add flavor to your food and are also full of healing antioxidants and phytonutrients. Better yet, they are fun to cook with, relatively inexpensive, and the history of culinary healing associated with herbs and spices spans centuries. They can also be used safely without setting off a neurological nightmare of headaches, muscle aches, and joint pain that can last for days.

Portion Distortion and Meal Timing

Our portion sizes have increased dramatically during the last forty years. Adults to-day consume an average of 300 more calories per day than they did in 1985. In the 1960s, the dinner plate measured an average of 8.5 inches. By comparison, today's dinner plate measures an average of 12 inches! That's nearly a 30 percent increase in size. The standard restaurant dinner plate has grown from 10 inches to 12 inches since 1970—a 20 percent increase. For a quick comparison, an 8-ounce cup of coffee with milk is about 45 calories. Today, your mocha latte is twice as big at 16 ounces, and with steamed milk and mocha syrup is 350 calories! If this is how you begin your day, it is a disaster for your metabolism and spurs chronic inflammation, pain, and weight gain.

How satisfied do you really feel after a meal? By the time you arrive to work after your morning latte and croissant, are you *hangry* (hungry and angry) and ready to rip into your nearest co-worker? If you feel hungry an hour after eating, something is seriously wrong. The last meal you ate should provide you with sustained energy for at least four to six hours. You should only eat three meals a day, and if you are active, you can have one snack. If you are experiencing the feelings of hunger, cravings, drowsiness, fatigue, mood swings, or an increase in pain, your meal was the problem. With the right combination of fats, protein, carbohydrates, vitamins, minerals, and phytonutrients, you will need less food on your plate and will remain fuller for longer stretches of time.

Each meal should contain protein, fats, and carbohydrates, keeping in mind the following serving sizes:

- **Clean protein:** 5 to 8 ounces, or about the size of a deck of playing cards
- **Healthy fat:** 2 to 3 servings of fat—healthy oils (olive and coconut), avocado, nuts or seeds, and especially the omega-3 fats found in protein.
- **Nonstarchy veggies:** 2 cups raw or 1 cup cooked. This should fill 50 percent of your plate or more.
- **Fiber-filled carbs:** ½ cup for women, ¾ cup for men. This should be less than 25 percent of your plate.

#2 Eat Whole Foods

Begin to incorporate as many whole foods as possible into your diet. Whole foods are foods that are unprocessed and unrefined, or processed and refined as little as possible, before being consumed. They typically do not contain added salt, sweeteners, or fat. These foods generally include whole grains; dark green, yellow, orange, red, and purple vegetables; fruits; legumes; nuts and seeds; unprocessed meat; and only if tolerated, dairy products from goats or sheep, as they are better tolerated and raised with fewer hormones and antibiotics. These whole foods contain high concentrations of antioxidants, such as polyphenols, fibers, and numerous other phytonutrients that may be protective against free radicals that cause chronic diseases.

Don't be fooled by labeling, as there is no legal labeling for a natural or whole food. The only legal label currently used is "USDA Certified Organic." This indicates that for plants no synthetic pesticides or fertilizers have been used, no genetically engineered seeds (GMOs), no sewage sludge and irradiation, and that they have been processed without adding artificial flavors, colors, or preservatives. For meat and animal products, it assures no use of added antibiotics or hormones and that the animals have been fed organic feed containing no animal by-products.

There is substantial evidence that eating a whole foods diet that includes quality protein, healthy fat, vegetables, and fruits is healthy and lowers your risk for certain diseases. The combined effects of vitamins, minerals, antioxidants, and phytonutrients are a powerful force that works to alleviate pain. Overall, whole foods offer:

- A greater nutrition source of more complex micronutrients
- An essential source of dietary fiber
- Access to naturally occurring protective substances, such as phytonutrients and antioxidants

Whole foods offer a wide range of benefits. Let's take a look at some specific healing foods to begin incorporating into your diet.

Protein

Protein helps stabilize blood sugar and should be included with each and every meal. Grass fed, free-range, hormone- and antibiotic-free cuts of lean meat—including lean cuts of chicken, turkey, beef, lamb, pork, and wild game—are part of the Healing Pain Diet.

Fats and Oils

Remember, the right fats are your friend and provide fatty acids needed for healing. Refrain from eating trans fats and stay away from saturated fats found in fatty cuts of meats. Choose olive and avocado oil instead of vegetable and corn oil, and consume avocados, olives, nuts, and coconut milk and oil. There are also healing natural fats found in fish and meat. Choose oily fish high in anti-inflammatory omega-3 fats and low in mercury, such as anchovies, herring, mackerel, salmon, sardines, and trout. Organic, free-range omega-3 eggs are also acceptable.

Nonstarchy Vegetables

This is a large part of what you will eat and will provide many of the anti-inflammatory phytonutrients and antioxidants. Vegetables, in particular, have the nutrients your cell's mitochondria require to help reduce inflammation and oxidative stress. The magic begins to happen when you consume nine servings per day. A serving is a cup of raw, leafy greens or ½ cup of cooked vegetables. Start consuming more leafy greens, such as kale, spinach, collards, dandelion greens, beet greens, mustard greens, radicchio, and arugula, plus garlic and onions.

Nuts and Seeds

Nuts and seeds make for a great snack when one is needed. They can also be used to decorate and add variety to a number of dishes. They pair well with salads and vegetables. Purchase only unsalted nuts that are not roasted in oil. Nut butters also make an excellent alternative and can be combined with fruits and vegetables, such as sliced apples, carrots, or celery. I recommend adding flaxseeds, chia seeds, hemp seeds, and unsalted mixed nuts to your diet. Peanuts should be strictly avoided for those with a known allergy and many find relief by avoiding them altogether.

Fruits

Fruits contain phytonutrients that have important anti-inflammatory properties, but you have to choose ones that are low on the glycemic index or glycemic load. These should be eaten one to two servings per day maximum and preferably with a meal that has a balance of fat and protein to help slow their sugar's absorption. I recommend incorporating more blueberries, strawberries, blackberries, raspberries, and pomegranate into your diet.

Grains and Legumes

Whole grains and legumes can be a great source of fiber, vitamins, and minerals and they aid digestion. The benefits include dietary fiber, several B vitamins (thiamine [B_1], riboflavin, niacin, and folate), and minerals (iron, magnesium, and selenium). Dietary fiber from whole grains or other foods may help reduce blood cholesterol levels and may lower risk of heart disease, high blood pressure, obesity, and type 2 diabetes. Remember, highly processed breads loaded with preservatives do not count as whole foods. Healthy options include whole oats, wild rice, quinoa, and beans. Because these foods help fill you up, they also help keep your weight in check.

What About My Vino?

Wine is often thought of as a superfood of the gods, and many popular media publications tout its beneficial effects as the masses rejoice and toast! Studies indicate that a 4-ounce glass of wine for men daily is healthy; women should drink one glass no more than four times a week, due to a link to the incidence of breast cancer. While phytonutrients, such as resveratrol, which can act as an anti-inflammatory, are present in red wine, remember that red wine is a form of sugar, although it does not raise blood sugar that much—joy! Furthermore, wine is excellent at lowering your inhibition for eating seconds and foods that are a one-way street toward weight gain and pain, so be careful. Alcohol mutes the sensors in your brain that signal when you have enough to eat.

#3 Choose Organic

Eating fresh produce is the best way to obtain the nutrients that support optimum health, but pesticides used on many crops remain a major health concern. Pesticides and herbicides make their way onto plants, into our soil, and into our waterways. By choosing organic foods, you can reap the health benefits of fresh food without exposing yourself and your family to potentially harmful chemicals. Pesticides present real health risks, particularly to children and those with health concerns. The toxicity most commonly associated with pesticides in animal studies includes disruptions in the normal functioning of the nervous and endocrine system. There are a few things you should be aware of and why they are important for your healing as you progress on the Healing Pain Diet.

Pesticides are toxic chemicals by design. They are created to kill living organisms—most commonly insects, plants, and fungi. Unfortunately, this makes its way from the factory farm into our food. Many pesticides pose significant health dangers to people. As acknowledged by US and international government agencies, different pesticides have been linked to a variety of health problems, including brain and nervous system toxicity and hormone disruption. Do you think something that is toxic to your nervous system can cause pain? You bet! And how about hormone disruption leading to increased weight gain? Pesticides are not something you should be ingesting by eating, drinking, or breathing them.

Dirty Dozen and Clean Fifteen

Every year, the Environmental Working Group (EWG) breaks down which fruits and vegetables have the most pesticides and which have the fewest. The EWG's mission is to make food supply more transparent so as to help you decide when it's worth spending extra for organic produce. If it works within your budget, the EWG recommends buying organic whenever possible. And if it's just not doable right now, the group's guide can help you make better choices. The EWG recommends that you eat more fruits and vegetables—even if you're exposed to pesticides—but now you'll have a better strategy. Use the following list, provided by the EWG, as a guide to better shopping choices when organic is not an option. Updates from the EWG can be found at http://www.ewg.org.

The Dirty Dozen: Fruits and Veggies with the *Most* Pesticides

- Strawberries
- Apples
- Nectarines
- Peaches
- Celery
- Grapes
- Cherries
- Spinach
- Tomatoes
- Sweet bell peppers
- Cherry tomatoes
- Cucumbers

The Clean Fifteen: Fruits and Veggies with the *Least* Pesticides

- Avocados
- Sweet corn
- Pineapples
- Cabbage
- Sweet peas (frozen)
- Onions
- Asparagus
- Mangoes
- Papayas
- Kiwi
- Eggplant
- Grapefruit
- Cantaloupe
- Cauliflower
- Honeydew melon

Soil Quality and Your Health

Plants extract nutrients from the soil and use them to thrive and grow. Animals, including us humans, then ingest the plants, hoping to benefit from nutrient density. Nutrient density is crucial to your healing as well as the promotion of overall health and prevention of disease. Therefore, the soil that plants are grown in is vital. Organic farmers have known for centuries that if you keep planting the same crop year after year without enriching the soil, crop yields will be less productive and the quality of the plant decreases. Modern agricultural methods have been successful at producing large amounts of food for the masses but have left our soil stripped of the essential nutrients we need in our food. Each successive generation of fast-growing, pest-resistant crop is truly less nutritious for you than the one before.

A landmark study on the topic by researchers from the University of Texas (UT) at Austin's Department of Chemistry and Biochemistry was published in December 2004 in the *Journal of the American College of Nutrition*. They studied US Department of Agriculture nutritional data from both 1950 and 1999 for forty-three different vegetables and fruits, finding "reliable declines" in the amount of protein, calcium, phosphorus, iron, vitamin B_2, and vitamin C over the past half century. There have likely been declines in other nutrients as well, such as magnesium, zinc, and vitamins B_6 and E, but they were not studied in 1950. Many of the vitamins and minerals mentioned are involved in the complex array of biochemical processes in your body, and a deficiency may lead to decreased healing. The most common nutrient deficiencies in the United States are vitamins A, C, D, E, and K as well as calcium, potassium, and magnesium. These vitamins and minerals support a healthy immune system and help with cell growth and repair, bone and muscle function, strength, and healing. The researchers compared this declining nutritional content to the current agricultural practices designed to improve traits (size, growth rate, pest resistance) other than nutrition. Soil quality is yet another reason to choose organic, so that you can ingest more of these healing vitamins and minerals.

#4 Consume a Rainbow of Phytonutrients and Antioxidants

Phytonutrients are plant compounds that have protective or disease preventive properties. Plants produce these chemicals to protect themselves, but recent research demonstrates that they can also protect humans against diseases. There are thousands of phytonutrients—and we still have much work to do discovering new ones and their benefits. Some of the well-known phytonutrients are lycopene in tomatoes and flavonoids in fruits. Each works differently. Most phytonutrients have antioxidant activity and protect our cells against oxidative damage and reduce the risk of developing certain types of cancer. Phytonutrients with antioxidant activity include: allyl sulfides (onions, leeks, garlic), carotenoids (fruits, carrots), flavonoids (fruits, vegetables), and polyphenols (tea, grapes). Indoles, which are found in cabbages, stimulate enzymes that make estrogen less effective and could reduce the risk for obesity and breast cancer. Other phytonutrients, such as terpenes (citrus fruits and cherries), contribute flavor, scent, and color. These substances are the building blocks for essential oils, have medicinal properties, and help in fighting bacteria, fungus, and environmental stress. The phytonutrient allicin, found in garlic, also has antibacterial properties. Some phytonutrients bind physically to cell walls, thereby preventing the adhesion of pathogens to human cell walls. Proanthocyanidins are responsible for the antiadhesion properties of cranberries.

Antioxidants are man-made or natural substances that may prevent or delay some types of cell damage. As natural substances, they are found in many whole foods, such as whole grains; dark green, yellow, orange, red, and purple vegetables; fruits; legumes; nuts; and seeds. Some antioxidants are produced by your body, but some are not. In addition, your body's natural antioxidant production can decline as you age. As man-made substances, antioxidants are available as dietary supplements or added to dietary supplements. Examples of antioxidants include beta-carotene, lutein, lycopene, glutathione, alpha lipoic acid, astaxanthin, resveratrol, vitamin C, and vitamin E.

Phytonutrient Healing Foods List

The following foods provide not only the vitamins and minerals to keep you healthy but also the phytonutrients and antioxidants necessary for cellular function. Each of these has its own unique anti-inflammatory, antibacterial, antimicrobial, and even anticancer properties. Many are necessary for proper hormonal, immune, gastrointestinal, and neuromusculoskeletal health. Begin incorporating them in large quantities into your diet during this phase—try to consume a rainbow of colors every day.

- **Red**: apples, beans, beets, bell peppers, blood oranges, cherries, cranberries, grapefruit, goji berries, grapes, onions, plums, pomegranate, radicchio, radishes, raspberries, rhubarb, strawberries, sweet red peppers, tomatoes
- **Orange:** apricots, bell peppers, cantaloupe, carrots, mangoes, nectarine, oranges, papayas, persimmons, pumpkin, squash, sweet potatoes, tangerines, turmeric, yams
- **Yellow:** apples, bananas, bell peppers, ginger, lemon, pears, pineapple, star fruit, summer squash
- **Green:** apples, artichokes, asparagus, avocados, bean sprouts, bell peppers, bitter melon, bok choy, broccoli, broccolini, brussels sprouts, cabbage, celery, cucumbers, green beans, green peas, green tea, salad greens (arugula, chard, Swiss chard, dandelion greens, kale, lettuce, mustard greens, spinach, turnip greens), limes, okra, olives, pears, snow peas, watercress, zucchini
- **Blue/black/purple:** bell peppers, berries (blueberries, blackberries, boysenberries, huckleberries), cabbage, carrots, cauliflower, eggplant, figs, grapes, kale, olives, plums, potatoes, prunes, rice
- **White/brown:** apples, cacao, cauliflower, coconut, coffee, dates, garlic, ginger, jicama, legumes, mushrooms, nuts (almonds, pecans, walnuts, Brazil), onions, pears, sauerkraut, seeds (flax, hemp, pumpkin, chia), shallots, tea, grains (wild rice, quinoa, oats)

#5 Increase Fiber and Fat

There is no doubt your current standard American diet is void of fiber, and it's completely sabotaging your fat-loss attempts and keeping you in a painful and toxic state. The average American barely reaches 14 grams of fiber per day, which is not even half the suggested daily recommended intake you should be receiving from your diet. As part of your core nutritional healing, it's important to ensure that you are adding enough fiber to your meals. Avoiding all processed foods will help to increase your overall fiber intake, because most processing of foods diminishes the natural fiber found in whole foods. If you are following the first four steps of core nutritional healing, you should already be getting more fiber in your diet.

Fiber comes in two forms: soluble and insoluble. They each have different benefits. Most of us are familiar with insoluble fiber, which acts to create movement in our digestive tract to help keep us regular. Regularity is essential, as each of us should have a bowel movement one to two times per day. Soluble fiber slows digestion and the release of carbohydrates into the bloodstream. This is important because it helps regulate blood sugar, control insulin levels, and prevent inflammation from rising. In addition to controlling insulin levels, soluble fiber also feeds the healthy bacteria in our gut, which acts to bolster our immune system. When you are healing, you will need all the help you can get.

Another important note often overlooked by clinicians is that fiber also traps toxins we may have ingested and prevents them from being absorbed or reabsorbed into the body. This is crucial to living in our toxic world. Fiber also keeps you fuller longer, because it is a form of carbohydrate your body is unable to digest. It creates a sensation of fullness without added calories. Fiber is found in plant-based foods, such as whole grains, nuts, legumes, vegetables, and fruits. Your goal should be a minimum of 30 grams daily, preferably working up toward 40 grams with a little bit of help and education.

In addition to fiber, it's important to ensure that you are adding plenty of healthy fats into your diet at this stage. Unfortunately, fat

The Ten Top Sources of Fiber

1. Blueberries
2. Raspberries
3. Avocados
4. Nuts
5. Seeds—especially chia and flaxseed
6. Beans
7. Broccoli
8. Kale
9. Apples
10. Cauliflower

gets a really bad reputation. It is also an easy target for misleading food labels, because the average consumer equates fat as something negative that will make you even fatter! The obesity epidemic really began right around the time of my birth, sometime between 1973 and 1980. Through a series of National Health Examination surveys, we know that obesity rates were still 14 percent until about 1980. Somewhere in the mid-1980s numbers began to rise toward 22 to 25 percent. That's known as the obesity epidemic, and there were two major changes occurring during that period. One, high-fructose corn syrup was introduced into our diet. Two, we began to embrace low-fat diets. Starting in 1977, the government began telling all Americans to eat less fat, and in the mid-1980s, we started producing low-fat products that in effect replaced the fat in our diet.

We went from being a country that ate about 40 percent of its calories in fat and 45 percent in carbohydrates to 34 percent fat and upward of 70 percent in carbohydrates. This was a dreadful mistake because the refined carbohydrates that replaced the fat are actually an efficient vehicle for chronic inflammation, insulin resistance, obesity, and pain. Fat primarily got its bad rap because of cardiovascular disease. Although saturated fats have been termed "bad fats," not all fats are created equal with respect to their effect on your body. Many people took the fat out of their diet and fat became feared. Eating too much saturated fat (animal fat, lard) and omega-6 fat (corn oil, soybean oil, vegetable oil) can have pro-inflammatory effects. But adding in fats high in omega-3 can have potent anti-inflammatory effects. Healthy fats can be found in fish, nuts, seeds, eggs, and certain oils, such as walnut, flaxseed, olive, and coconut.

Friends or Food Foes?

Much of your success (or failure) begins with your social circle. Food is a major social event in our society and, for many, food equals friendship, family, and love. But what if the friends and family that surround you are unaware of or unsupportive of the changes you are trying to make? For many people, telling them you are no longer eating at the not-so-healthy restaurant you frequented or that you purchase organic

General Guidelines for Getting Started

Healing begins by eating real, whole foods. If most of your meals are packaged, processed, frozen, or boxed, chances are you are not getting what you need in the way of nutrition.

Aim for nine servings of plant foods daily. A typical serving is ½ cup of cooked vegetable, one cup of raw leafy vegetable, or a medium-size piece of fruit (once or twice daily). Aim for three servings at every meal of plant foods, so that you will make the requirement within the three meals a day.

Make a protein shake for breakfast. Many people either skip breakfast or have dessert for breakfast (a bagel, doughnut, or other sugary concoction). These types of foods raise blood sugar, spike insulin, and start off your day on the wrong foot. What can you eat for breakfast? A healing protein shake is a great way to start your day and can be combined with some healthy fat from coconut or almond milk and blueberries for a delicious and easy morning routine. Meal replacement shakes in the morning are my number one strategy for fat loss: Start your day with a healing protein shake!

Eat a variety of rainbow-colored foods. Each of your meals should have a variety of color. If your meals run from the white to beige range, you are eating all the wrong foods. The biggest time for error is in the morning, where it's easy to grab a breakfast pastry, bagel, or toast, or quickly eat a bowl of cereal before you rush out the door. However, if you started the day with a protein-infused fruit smoothie with mixed berries (blueberries, raspberries, strawberries), you would begin the day with more energy.

Eat by the clock. That means eat within an hour of waking up. Spread out your meals every four to six hours and only eat three meals a day. Your last meal should be three hours before you go to bed, so that you are not sleeping with a belly full of food. While you sleep your energy should go toward restoration, not digesting food.

Choose organic whenever possible. Organic foods contain more of the nutrients your body needs and none of the harmful pesticides or hormones.

foods can be a lot to digest. Quite often I find myself coaching clients on their interpersonal relationships and how they relate to your health. We can focus on the food, but some of you may receive the greatest benefit by eliminating toxic people from your dining table. Learning to put your needs and health forward as a priority is often the first step you need to take. This may mean e-mailing your closest group of friends and letting them know you will be making some changes to your diet over the next thirty days and would like their support.

According to one study, participants who enrolled in a weight-loss program with friends did a better job of keeping off their weight. In teaming up with friends, these enrollees were given social support in addition to standard treatment. Two thirds of those who enrolled with friends had kept off their weight six months after the meetings ended. In contrast, only a quarter of those who attended on their own had achieved that same success. Online social networks are fast becoming a way for like-minded seekers of health to connect and have helped with social support for weight loss. Join the Healing Pain Program support group by visiting www.drjoetatta.com/group.

Dr. Joe's Top Healing Foods Checklist

All leafy greens
Almonds
Avocados
Basil
Blueberries and blackberries
Bone broth
Coconut oil
Coconut yogurt
Cruciferous vegetables
    (broccoli, cauliflower,
    brussels sprouts, kale)

Extra-virgin olive oil
Ginger
Grass-fed beef
Green tea
Oregano
Pomegranate
Rosemary
Spinach
Thyme
Turmeric
Wild-caught salmon

Food Shopping List

Clean Lean Animal Protein
(preferably organic, grass-fed or wild-caught)

Beef
Chicken
Lamb
Pork
Sausage with no additives,
    preservatives, nitrites,
    nitrates, gluten, or MSG

Turkey
Veal
Wild game (venison, rabbit,
    pheasant, quail)

Fish and Shellfish (* indicates high in omega-3s):

Anchovies*

Clams*

Cod

Crab

Halibut*

Herring*

Lobster

Mackerel*

Mussels*

Oysters*

Salmon*

Sardines*

Scallops

Shrimp

Trout*

Nuts, Seeds, and Nut Butters

Almonds

Brazil nuts

Chia seeds

Flaxseeds

Hazelnuts

Peanuts (technically a legume
and allergenic)

Pumpkin seeds

Sesame seeds

Sunflower seeds

Walnuts

Note: Avoid any nuts or seeds
that cause allergy.

Fiber-Filled Carbs

Apples

Beans (black, white, red,
green, lima, and chickpeas)

Beets

Berries

Brown rice

Lentils

Peas (split, black-eyed, green)

Quinoa

Quinoa pasta

Squash

Sweet potatoes

Nonstarchy Vegetables

Arugula

Asparagus

Beet greens

Bok choy

Broccoli

Broccolini

Brussels sprouts

Cauliflower

Chard

Chicory

Cilantro

Collard greens

Dandelion greens

Endive

Escarole

Kale

Lettuce greens   Radish leaves
Mizuna   Red onions
Mushrooms   Romaine lettuce
Mustard greens   Spinach
Parsley   Watercress
Radicchio

Oil for Cooking

Coconut oil   Olive oil (only for low-medium
Ghee (clarified butter)   flame sautéing)

Oil for Dressing (Preferably organic, virgin, cold-pressed—*not to be heated!*)

Avocado oil   Hemp oil
Extra-virgin olive oil   Walnut oil
Flax oil

Fermented Foods

Lacto-fermented carrots, ginger, cabbage, sauerkraut,
    coconut kefir

Beverages

Coffee   Sparkling water
Herbal tea   Tea
Naturally flavored waters   Water

Now you have the foundation for a healthy start to core nutritional healing. If you follow this plan for three weeks, eliminating processed foods and pesticides and instead incorporating low-glycemic, organic whole foods in a rainbow of colors, healthy fats, and fiber, you should notice a decrease in your pain within three weeks and an average weight loss of 7 to 10 pounds. In the next chapter, we'll explore the gut-joint connection and the top five foods to eliminate from your diet in order to heal your gut and lower your inflammation. For more information on how food can alleviate your pain and to download healthy recipes, visit www.drjoetatta.com/thehealingpaindiet.

Dr. Joe's Pain Relief Reminders

- Start off your day with a healing protein shake for breakfast.
- Consume more omega-3 fatty acids (found in fish, grass-fed beef, nuts, seeds) and less omega-6 fatty acids (found in vegetable oil, corn oil, and soybean oil), and add more fiber to your diet.
- Eliminate processed foods, food additives such as MSG, preservatives, and artificial sweeteners.
- Eat organic foods as much as possible—especially with regard to the Dirty Dozen.
- Focus on eating whole foods, in a rainbow of colors, which are rich in fiber, phytonutrients, and antioxidants.

6

GUT HEALING

The Basics of Gut Healing

Time frame: Three weeks to heal a leaky gut and decrease inflammation, autoimmunity, and pain.

Changes: Eliminate gluten, all dairy, sugar, GMOs (corn and soy), and eggs.

Supportive supplementation: Follow the 4R gut-healing supplement protocol.

Prepare for success: Download the complete shopping guide, 7-day gut-healing meal plan, and recipes, all available at www.drjoetatta.com/thehealingpaindiet.

Results: Alleviation of six more points on a pain scale and accompanied by 7 to 10 pounds of weight loss in three weeks. Many are pain-free by the end of three weeks.

Pain is a master at concealing its true identity. It draws your attention to one area, distracting you from the real origin of your pain. In the Healing Pain Program, we are going to get to the root cause of your pain. But to do that we have to unearth exactly where the inflammation in your body is truly beginning. You may feel that your pain begins and ends in your joints or muscles, but in reality it often begins in your gut.

In the Core Nutrition Program, we worked on improving the essential fatty acids, vitamins, minerals, phytonutrients, fiber, and antioxidants necessary to begin to support a healthy immune system and reverse chronic inflammation so that you can lose weight and alleviate pain. We also spoke about some essential lifestyle habits to begin or improve upon. In my experience, the core nutrition program is an entry point, but the real magic occurs in the gut-healing protocol outlined in this chapter. If you continue to struggle with pain from such conditions as diabetes, an autoimmune disease, arthritis, neu-romuscular disease, or chronic unrelenting joint pain, implementing the gut-healing phase is your next step. Three weeks on this protocol has changed the lives of many. In the gut-healing stage of the Heal-ing Pain Program, we'll explore how your immune system gets out of balance and causes low-grade but persistent inflammation and how eliminating certain foods can heal your gut—and your pain.

Eliminating your pain as well as inches around your waist is totally worth the challenge. After the gut-healing stage, many people feel so good they continue to eat this way! Preparing yourself for the change is most of the battle, so make sure to purge your kitchen of the five foods to eliminate (see page 113) and use the shopping guide and food list from Chapter 5 to stock up on foods you can eat and use to pre-pare your meals. It is important that you eliminate the five foods for a minimum of three weeks, as a shorter time period will not enable your leaky gut to heal and immune system to calm. If you have struggled with a severe autoimmune disease, it may take as long as three months to achieve the result you desire, but you will definitely notice a mea-surable change within three weeks. Eat only the foods that are allowed on the Healing Pain Program.

Your Gut, Home of Your Immune System

Inflammation is present if there is pain, and it is associated with many chronic diseases you struggle with today. Most people think of their immune system as cells floating around in their bloodstream that at-tack a virus or bacteria when they are sick. What most people don't realize is that the majority of their immune system lives in their *gut*. Even many health-care practitioners do not know that 70 percent of your immune system is located in your digestive tract, making a healthy gut a major focal point if you want to maintain optimal health. Why is the majority of your immune system located in your gut? Be-cause the first wave of attack from foreign invaders, such as bacteria, fungi, viruses, toxins, and even food particles you are allergic to or have an intolerance to, happens in your gut. This is where your first line of defense occurs. The gastrointestinal tract's immune system is referred to as gut-associated lymphoid tissue (GALT) and works to protect the body from invasion. To fend off foreign invaders, your immune system lines the wall of your intestine with specialized cells. If not stopped by your immune system, these foreign invaders can easily enter your body, passing through weak points in your intestinal wall and gaining access to your bloodstream, where they can circulate around your body and cause harm.

The days of looking at the digestive tract as a passive tube where food enters, is "digested," and exits is an outdated and simplistic view of how nutrition affects your overall health. Any discussion of the digestive tract must include not only the food but also the effect food is having on your immune health. A healthy and robust immune system is your number one defense system against inflammation, pain, and obesity—the link to all disease. The root of your pain and weight gain is inflammation, and it begins in your gut.

The combination of an altered microbiome, food intolerances, leaky gut, and other lifestyle effects discussed in the Healing Pain Program leads to the production and exacerbation of many symptoms throughout the body. This initiates a cascade of physical changes and results in a variety of symptoms that quite often don't fit into our current medical system's diagnostic labels. Pain and obesity are good examples of this, and now that you're reading this book, you will finally be able to connect the dots in places where practitioners have often given you blank stares or failed treatments. Proper food choices will decrease inflammation, heal your gut, and promote the regrowth of a healthy microbiome. Just like your lawn, which needs to be fertilized and reseeded in certain areas that have become barren for whatever reason, the Healing Pain Program will teach you how to cultivate a healthy microbiome.

The Microbiome and Immunity

The microbiome is the name for the more than 100 trillion bacteria that live on and in our body. Overall, the number of bacteria in the gut is tenfold greater than the number of cells in the human body. More than five hundred species and more than 100 trillion bacteria coexist and have coevolved with humans. You are more microbiome than you are human. This symbiotic relationship in our gut exists to provide the positive health effects of producing B vitamins, vitamin K, and short-chain fatty acids; lowering pH; producing anti-microbial compounds; and modulating the immune system.

Because 70 percent of the cells that make up the body's immune system exist in the lining of our intestinal tract, the microbiome assists in immune-related responses. The majority lives within our gut but also inhabits other mucous membranes, such as in the sinus cavities, on our skin, and in the urogenital areas. Much of the recent research reveals that the microbiome has some surprising effects on our physiology. Each of us has a unique personal microbiome. For the most part we have a symbiotic relationship with these microbes. They help us break down and digest food, produce nutrients that we absorb, defend us from viruses and harmful bacteria, and support our immunity.

The Gut-Joint Connection

Hippocrates, the father of modern medicine, stated that all healing begins in the gut. There is a symbiotic relationship regarding our health and the microbiome of our intestinal tract. Diet plays a crucial role in maintaining the delicate balance of our microbiome and the proper amount and type of bacteria, fungi, and viruses, as well as avoiding organ failure. When alterations of our microbiome are compromised, dysbiosis occurs, meaning that there is a microbial imbalance, which can lead to a variety of illnesses from inflammatory bowel disease to cancer. This is not only observed in the gut but also in parts of the body where no direct anatomical connection exists. This new area of science is beginning to identify "gut-related axes," such as the gut-brain axis. Of particular interest is the existence of a gut-joint axis and its relation to musculoskeletal pain.

Regarding diet, a relationship between obesity, inflammation, and the gut microbiome has also been established. Obesity is a disorder of chronic low-grade inflammation and has been implicated in dysbiosis. Microbiome changes in the gastrointestinal tract can have multiple effects; however, the primary considerations causing inflammation are:

- Overabsorption of bacterial cellular debris
- Nutrient malabsorption
- Intestinal permeability or leaky gut, where the lining becomes permeable to antigens.

The passage of antigenic material (toxins, bacteria, food antibodies/allergies, and microbes) through the lining of your gut and into circulation can deposit them in your joints, tendons, synovial sheaths, muscles, and ligaments. The link between obesity, inflammation, and our microbiome is beginning to reveal how previously thought chronic musculoskeletal problems, such as osteoarthritis, are not simply one of physical wear and tear. This may explain why a large number of obese patients develop osteoarthritis in non-weight-bearing joints, such as the wrist joints, pointing to a systemic inflammatory cause. The condition and function of the gastrointestinal (GI) tract are essential to our well-being.

After the respiratory tract, the GI tract constitutes the second-largest body surface area, consisting of the stomach and intestines. It is important for overall health but also poses an enormous threat to the integrity of the whole body during the digestive process. It is not surprising, therefore, that this organ is often affected by inflammatory diseases. The continuous challenges to the GI surfaces might explain why most of the surface cells have a rapid turnover; most are replaced after three to four days. Furthermore, the surface is protected by large quantities of essential secretions, from saliva in the oral cavity to colonic secretion in the large bowel. These secretions contain factors of great importance for the lubrication of the mucosa and for functions of the GI tract but also hundreds of significant ingredients for protecting our immunity. They are extremely sensitive to foreign chemicals. About 50 percent of the two thousand pharmaceutical drugs registered in Sweden have reported GI side effects: for example, dry mouth, nausea, vomiting, diarrhea, and constipation. Ultimately, when the microbiome is compromised either from drugs or food, and you develop leaky gut, toxic materials begin to pass through your digestive wall and into your body, where they are seen as foreign invaders, initiating an immune response of inflammation and joint pain.

Do You Have a Leaky Gut?

Your gut is a unique barrier between the inside of your body and the outside world—its job is to allow important nutrients inside the body while keeping out everything else. This makes it a highly selective, semipermeable barrier. The inner lining of your intestines closely controls what is absorbed and allowed to pass through. Maintaining the integrity of this barrier is crucial. The inner lining of your gut wall is one cell thick. These single-celled warriors stand side by side, forming what is known as a tight junction. Nothing is able to pass in between these single cells, unless it is a vitamin, mineral, or a food particle that has been thoroughly digested and broken down into the smallest possible size. When you are healthy, your gut is sealed tight from foreign invaders, such as bacteria, toxins, and large undigested food particles.

When these tight junctions begin to break down, the one-cell-thick barrier of your gut becomes inflamed and develops holes that begin allowing for the passage of bacteria, toxins, and undigested food particles that normally are too large to pass. And worse, with the lining of your intestine inflamed, it is unable to perform the crucial job of absorbing nutrients. You have a double blow of not allowing the good to be absorbed, while the bad barge on through. Although the technical name for this is intestinal permeability, most of us now refer to it as leaky gut syndrome. Leaky gut is a condition whereby toxic food particles, environmental chemicals, and bacteria leak through your digestive tract and enter your body.

Mainstream medical practitioners generally do not recognize leaky gut as a contributing factor to disease and illness, but once you heal it, you will be amazed at the far-reaching beneficial health effects of tightly sealing your gut. Leaky gut is most readily associated with the signs and symptoms of irritable bowel syndrome, such as constipation, diarrhea, indigestion, nausea, gas, cramping, or discomfort. Many with a leaky

LEAKY GUT

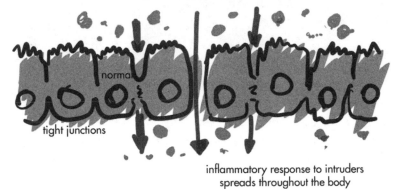

undigested food particles/ toxins

normal

tight junctions

inflammatory response to intruders
spreads throughout the body

gut may experience these symptoms initially; however, if not resolved, the chronic systemic inflammation it causes can have a far-reaching effect in other parts of the body. Some of the major symptoms of chronic leaky gut include joint and muscle pain, headaches, mood swings, eczema, weight gain, and fatigue. Many of these symptoms occur together simultaneously, and a traditional medical professional may have a difficult time diagnosing the condition, because multiple systems and organs in your body are affected at the same time. It's the perfect storm. How does this happen? Once food particles, bacteria, and toxins are allowed to pass through and into your bloodstream, your immune

Seven Signs That You Have a Leaky Gut

- Digestive issues (bloating, gas, diarrhea, constipation, or irritable bowel syndrome)
- Seasonal allergies or asthma
- Autoimmune diseases, such as celiac disease, psoriasis, lupus, or rheumatoid arthritis
- Chronic joint and muscle pain or fatigue
- Mood issues, including depression, anxiety, ADD/ADHD
- Acne, rosacea, eczema
- Food allergies and intolerances

system launches an attack and begins the inflammatory process. If this occurred just one time, it would not be a big deal. But if you have had a leaky gut for a long time, this has perpetuated a chronic inflammatory environment.

Leaky Gut and Your Pain

When foreign invaders pass through a leaky gut and enter the bloodstream, they are known as an antigen, which is basically a foreign substance that induces an immune response in the body. In return, your immune system creates antibodies to attack and destroy the foreign invaders (antigens), such as bacteria, viruses, or undigested food particles or proteins. The antibody will bind with the antigen in an attempt to render it harmless. This binding of antigen and antibody is called an immune complex. However, with a persistent leaky gut, there is an overproduction of immune complexes, which can act like antigens of their own and may cause chronic systemic inflammation. These immune complexes circulate around the body and are deposited in various tissues and organs. Now when I say *organ*, most people think of the heart, liver, or kidneys. However, most fail to recognize that the largest organ in the body is skeletal muscle! Many of these immune complexes are deposited in the joints, muscles, synovial membranes, and tendons throughout the musculoskeletal system. Once deposited in tissues, they cause yet another local inflammatory response. At times the immune system can even attack the body's own cells, tissues, and organs. The immune complexes can set off inflammation in any joint or muscle, which will cause pain, swelling, and stiffness. When this occurs, you unknowingly may believe the problem is localized to a specific joint or joints. Now you know the root cause of your inflammation actually stems from your gut!

Leaky Gut and Autoimmune Disease

Leaky gut or intestinal permeability is also a critical factor when it comes to the approximately 50 million Americans who suffer with an autoimmune disease. One in twelve Americans—and one in nine women—will develop an autoimmune disorder. And since it is clear that not every patient with an autoimmune disease is correctly diagnosed, the prevalence is certainly higher than that, with women suffering more than men. There are more than eighty different types of autoimmune diseases. Many of them have similar symptoms, which makes them extremely difficult to diagnose, and upward of 15 percent of Americans have more than one autoimmune disease at the same time.

There are three factors that are needed for autoimmunity to develop: (1) a genetic predisposition, (2) a trigger, and (3) leaky gut. You need all three; just having one, such as a genetic predisposition, is not enough. Something must trigger a gene to express an autoimmune disease. A poor diet can be enough of a trigger to cause leaky gut and turn on a gene for autoimmunity, which leads to pain. If you have a leaky gut, you may be on a continuum of autoimmunity, with either subtle symptoms or more than one autoimmune disease to battle. By sealing your leaky gut, you will put out the fire that feeds your inflammation, calm your immune system, and decrease your pain. The best part is you can do all of this naturally—through diet without the side effects of drugs or surgery—and learn the simple lessons of self-healing that will last a lifetime.

Contributors to a Leaky Gut

- Alcohol
- Corticosteroids
- Stress
- Sugar
- Food intolerance and allergies
- Overtraining or endurance exercise
- Infections
- Toxins
- Genetic predisposition
- NSAIDs
- Nutrient deficiencies
- Caffeine
- Yeast overgrowth
- Antibiotics

Are You Allergic—or Sensitive?

There is a difference between a food allergy and a food sensitivity or intolerance. You may understand the concept of a food allergy if you have been around children who are allergic to peanuts, one of the most prevalent allergens. A food allergy is most commonly seen as an immediate immune reaction to a specific food each and every time you eat it. Your immune system identifies the particular food as foreign and attacks it. As with most immune reactions, proteins in a food are often the culprit. Reactions can range from mild to severe, including the potentially life-threatening condition known as anaphylaxis, where your throat can close up and you can no longer breathe. In the United States food allergy symptoms send someone to the emergency room every three minutes. Other symptoms of an acute food allergy may include a rash, severe gastrointestinal disturbances, and cardiovascular problems. Symptoms typically appear within minutes to an hour after eating the food to which you are allergic. Many are aware of food allergies causing anaphylaxis (the most common example being peanuts and kids), but they may also experience milder symptoms, such as itchy lips/tongue/throat, stuffy nose, headaches, belly ache, diarrhea, gas, bloating, skin reactions, and sudden fatigue. Identifying a food allergy is typically performed with a blood test; however, most adults have their "trigger food" figured out because the reaction is so quick.

A nonimmediate, or delayed, response to a food is what is known as an intolerance or food sensitivity. This differs from an immediate food allergy response in that symptoms may not appear for hours or days, making it difficult to pinpoint exactly which foods are causing what reaction in the body, especially since people tend to eat the same foods over and over. Because of this, food intolerances often remain hidden. For years people continue to eat and expose themselves to the same irritating food day after day, causing inflammation, dysbiosis, and leaky gut to develop. This combination leads to systemic inflammation that has far-reaching effects, causing weight gain and pain. Symptoms of food intolerances or sensitivities include congestion, headaches, stomach pain, constipation, diarrhea, gas, bloating, foggy head, and skin issues. Weight gain, fatigue, joint pain, tendinitis, muscle pain, and depression are some of the most misdiagnosed and difficult to detect because our medical community is often busy treating symptoms. If you suspect you may have a food sensitivity or intolerance, you can be tested by a functional medicine practitioner. Later in the chapter, you'll also begin to eliminate certain foods that are often the prime suspects in causing food sensitivities, so you will have a better understanding of how particular foods affect your overall health and how you feel.

Your 4R Gut-Healing Protocol

Jessica was struggling with irritable bowel syndrome (IBS) and chronic back pain. The notion that her IBS could be the cause of her back pain was comforting, since she had seen almost every specialist and still could not find relief. I explained that a simple four-step process could alleviate both her stomach and back pain.

The same process could work for you. Even though each step is happening simultaneously, I have broken them down for you to help you better understand what is going on in your body. A properly functioning digestive system is where your healing begins. In functional medicine we use a program that goes by the simple acronym of the "4Rs": remove, replace, repopulate, and repair. The 4R program can lead to dramatic improvement in your symptoms, and sometimes even complete resolution.

#1 Remove

First, we begin by removing and eliminating anything that can negatively affect the environment of the GI tract, including food allergens, parasites, and problematic bacteria or yeast. Allowing these foods and bacteria into your bloodstream is causing a continual immune response, keeping inflammation steady and not allowing pain to subside or weight to be lost despite all good intentions. By removing just five foods, not only will we repair your gut, but also this is often the first step in ridding your body of microorganisms, such as bacteria, viruses, fungi, parasites, yeast, and toxins that are overpopulated and causing your microbiome to be in a dysbiotic state. Gluten, dairy, and sugar are the top three foods to remove, along with genetically modified organisms (GMOs) and eggs.

#2 Replace

Your digestive system doesn't absorb food; it absorbs nutrients. Throughout your digestive tract, enzymes are secreted that break down fats, protein, and carbohydrates into their smallest form, so they can be easily digested and absorbed by your gut. Many factors can reduce the amount of enzymes, thus making digestion and nutrient absorption challenging—if not impossible. If we don't have enough digestive enzymes, we can't break down our food—which means even though we're eating well, we aren't absorbing all that good nutrition. Fewer enzymes are produced as we age and are vital for those over the age of sixty-five, but enzymes can also decrease by other factors, including intestinal inflammation caused by leaky gut, food allergies, and intolerances, low stomach acid, dysbiosis, medications, and disease. And let's not forget stress! Daily stress and the fight-or-flight response impairs the secretion of digestive enzymes, which is one of the reasons why so many people have a difficult time digesting food if they

SIBO: The First Buggers to Go!

Small intestinal bacterial overgrowth (SIBO) occurs when bacteria and/or yeast invade and overpopulate the sterile environment of the small intestine, a place where relatively few organisms live. The small intestine is normally sterile because bacteria are killed by strong pancreatic or stomach enzymes. When an overgrowth of bacteria and/or yeast occurs, it may have severe metabolic consequences. This overgrowth is the reason many struggle with symptoms of irritable bowel syndrome (IBS), such as gas, bloating, abdominal pain, and discomfort. You can pretty much bet the house that if you struggle with IBS, SIBO is one of the underlying causes. One study in the *American Journal of Gastroenterology* revealed that upward of 78 percent of patients with IBS also tested positive for SIBO. In other words, their intestines were overrun with bad bugs! Given that gut issues can have far-reaching effects outside your belly, SIBO can be a contributing factor to the production of your pain. A 2001 study in the *Journal of Musculoskeletal Pain* revealed that small intestine bacterial overgrowth is associated with fibromyalgia and that eradicating SIBO alleviated symptoms in patients suffering with fibromyalgia. Killing the bad bugs and helping the good bugs to flourish is what the 4R program is all about!

are stressed or anxious. Replacing digestive enzymes or aiding those that are already present will help you digest your food and extract the essential nutrients. Consuming digestive enzymes, such as protease, lipase, amylase, and betaine HCl, prior to eating a meal will aid in digestion and absorption of vitamins, minerals, and nutrients. Natural digestive bitters made from dandelion, fennel, or ginger can also help.

#3 Repopulate

The more than five hundred different species of microorganisms that reside in your gut can profoundly influence your overall health. The third step of the 4R program introduces probiotics (a.k.a. good, or friendly, bacteria) to reestablish a healthy microbiome. Probiotics are beneficial microorganisms found in the gut. Frequent rounds of strong antibiotics throughout your life can kill both good and bad bacteria, causing dysbiosis in your microbiome. Probiotics serve many functions, but perhaps the most important is to fend off the bad bacteria and pathogens. They do this by competing with them for space in your gut, secreting antimicrobial substances to kill them, and competing for nutrients.

You can absolutely alter and influence your microbiome to flourish by eating probiotic foods or supplements that contain the "good" bacteria—these include such species as bifidobacterium, lactobacillus, and *Saccharomyces boulardi*. Probiotics in the form of supplements or food are often needed to help reestablish a balanced gut microbiome. Fermented foods, such as coconut yogurt, kefir, and sauerkraut, are good sources of probiotics. In addition, these friendly bacteria can be boosted by feeding them prebiotics.

Prebiotics are a special form of dietary fiber that acts as a fertilizer for the good bacteria in your gut. They are food ingredients that selectively stimulate the growth of beneficial microorganisms already in the colon. In other words, prebiotics are the food probiotics thrive on. Prebiotics include fructans, inulin, arabinoagalactans, and fructooligosaccharides. These are found in such foods as artichokes, garlic, leeks, onions, and chicory. Flaxseeds and beans are also good sources of prebiotics. By eating the right foods, such as asparagus, spinach, artichokes, Jerusalem artichokes, onions, leeks, garlic, and flaxseeds, you can the repopulate the good bacteria and heal your gut.

#4 Repair

It's also important to repair your leaky gut. Repair provides the nutritional support for the regeneration and healing of your gastrointestinal tract by supplying key nutrients that can often be in short supply in a compromised leaky gut. Repair is necessary to heal from the waves of inflammation in your gut and restore the semipermeable barrier that keeps the foreign invaders out but allows the good nutrition to filter through. Nutritional support for the lining of your gut is achieved directly through food as well as supplements critical for the structure and function of the gut wall. For repair and healing, the amino acids L-glutamine and arginine, and vitamins B_5 (pantothenic acid) and D are needed. Fish oil, which contains EPA and DHA, has also been shown to decrease inflammation in the gut and heal the intestinal lining.

The Five Foods to Eliminate

To rebalance your microbiome and alleviate the symptoms of leaky gut that are causing you to be in pain and overweight, it's important to eliminate certain inflammatory foods from your diet. The biggest culprits are gluten, dairy, sugar, GMOs (especially soy and corn), and eggs.

I recommend eliminating all five foods to fight pain for three weeks, in addition to adding some supplements to assist in healing your gut. If any food is one of the five foods, then don't eat it during this entire period. This will give your body the time it needs to heal from the ravages of years of leaky gut symptoms, rebalance your microbiome, and allow your immune system to stop the process of chronic inflammation. Any shorter than three weeks will not allow your gut to heal, immune system to quiet down, and microbiome to rebalance. Your body needs time to clear and detoxify from foods that your immune system has overreacted to for years, causing inflammation, pain, and weight gain.

You may see a few symptoms worsen in the first three to four days, as your body adjusts. Such symptoms rarely last more than two days; some of the more common ones include fatigue and headaches. This is only temporary and not everyone experiences these symptoms. Waiting on the other side is a pain-free and lighter you, able to enjoy life without being burdened by symptoms.

Much of the joint pain, tightness, tension, aches, and weight gain that you have struggled with for years, and that has not responded to conventional medical therapy, will be resolved after removing the five foods from your diet. After a few days, you will see your symptoms start to lessen and disappear. You are reducing the burden your immune system has had to deal with for years, from fighting the armies of invaders due to leaky gut and microbiome imbalances. Removing these foods will allow your body to heal and begin to function efficiently again. You may just wake up one day and notice that your fingers feel less stiff; your knees, back, and hips don't ache; and your neck pain and headaches disappear. By the end of three weeks, you will recognize improvement in many symptoms, including decreased pain, weight loss, increased energy, increased mental focus, decreased GI symptoms, and a sense of overall vitality.

Gluten's Gotta Go

If you have pain, gluten is the first item that needs to be completely eliminated from your diet. Gliadin is the protein found in wheat, rye, and barley that many people are sensitive to or that causes an outright autoimmune reaction when they consume these products. Your immune system sees gluten as the enemy and will unleash weapons to attack it, causing inflammation not only in your gut but also in other organs and tissues.

Celiac disease is a genetic autoimmune disease that damages the microscopic fingerlike projections in the small intestine called villi. The resultant inflammation of the villi interferes with absorption of nutrients from food. An estimated 1 in 133 Americans, or about 1 percent of the population, has celiac disease. It can affect men and women across all ages and races. Many people remain undiagnosed or are misdiagnosed with irritable bowel syndrome. Celiac disease can lead to a number of other disorders, including infertility, reduced bone density, neurological disorders, some cancers, and other autoimmune diseases. The only solution for someone with celiac disease is a completely gluten-free diet. Even the smallest amounts of gluten can make a person very ill. Checking for celiac disease through a biopsy of intestinal tissue or genetic testing is of the utmost importance for anyone who has an autoimmune disease. Interestingly, a number of people with celiac disease don't experience classic gut problems, and even those with severe intestinal damage can present with no symptoms at all. This can make a diagnosis difficult, often taking years to discover.

Not all people who react negatively to gluten actually have celiac disease, but the symptoms of gluten sensitivity are similar. Nonceliac gluten sensitivity exists in upward of 40 percent of people. These people still experience side effects when they eat gluten but may test negative for celiac disease antibodies. The idea that gluten sensitivity is regarded as principally a disease of the intestine is a misconception. A 2015 study in the *Annals of Nutrition and Metabolism* cited the most common nonintestinal symptoms of nonceliac gluten sensitivity: brain fog; headaches; fatigue; bone, muscle, and joint pain; leg or arm numbness; skin rashes; and depression. A 2016 paper in the *Journal of Clinical Rheumatology* supported the hypothesis of nonceliac gluten sensitivity and its association with fibromyalgia, spondyloarthritis, and various autoimmune conditions. Gluten not only affects your musculoskeletal system and creates pain but it also triggers many neurological problems. Gluten ataxia occurs when the antibodies that are produced in response to the ingestion of gluten attack a part of your brain called the cerebellum. Your cerebellum is the part of your brain that controls balance and coordination. Gluten ataxia can present with hard-to-diagnose balance problems, gait abnormalities, and incoordination. Peripheral neuropathy is another neurological side effect of gluten, causing pain, numbness, and tingling in the extremities of hands and feet.

Gluten is the greatest offender of a leaky gut. The gluten molecule triggers zonulin, a protein that causes tight junctions to loosen, producing increased intestinal permeability (leaky gut). As you repeatedly subject your gut to gluten, more and more of these tight junctions loosen, causing the passage of bacteria, food antigens, and other foreign invaders through your intestinal wall. Once through the delicate intestinal lining, a chronic low-grade inflammatory environment begins.

Gluten is found in the following grains: wheat, including such varieties as spelt, kamut, farro, durum, bulgur, and semolina; barley; rye; and triticale. Note: Oats do not contain gluten; however, almost all oat products on the market are cross-contaminated with gluten-containing grains during factory processing and packaging. Unless the oats label specifically says "processed in a facility that does not process grain," consider it contaminated with gluten.

Non-gluten grains include amaranth, buckwheat, millet, oats (see note above), quinoa (a seed), rice, wild rice, sorghum, and teff.

Symptoms of Nonceliac Gluten Sensitivity

Gut Symptoms	Systemic Symptoms
Bloating	Fatigue
Abdominal pain	Bone pain
Diarrhea	Muscle pain
Constipation	Joint pain
Gas	Ataxia
GERD (gastroesophageal reflux)	Numbness
Nausea	Loss of balance
	Skin rashes or dermatitis
	Weight gain
	Depression
	ADD/ADHD

Ditch the Dairy

Most of us have been raised and almost brainwashed to believe that we need dairy products to grow up big and strong and that it's even more important as we age. An entire industry has developed around

What Contains Gluten?

While some foods clearly contain gluten, it may be hiding in places you don't suspect. The following lists will help you determine where gluten may be present in your foods.

More Obvious Sources of Gluten (wheat and grain products)

Bread crumbs/panko
Bread, including corn bread and
    breaded foods
Cakes
Cereals
Cookies
Couscous
Crackers

Dumplings
Muffins
Oats (by contamination)
Pancakes
Pasta, noodles
Pastries and doughnuts
Pies/piecrusts
Waffles

Hidden Sources of Gluten

Beef, chicken, and vegetable stock
    (unless specified as gluten-free)
    as well as bouillon cubes
Beer
Candy
Condiments, such as ketchup and
    barbecue sauce
Gravy
Lunch meats and cold cuts

Matzos
Packaged mixes
Soufflés
Soy sauce
Tamari
Vegan meat substitutes, such as
    seitan
Wheat germ, wheat bran, and
    wheatgrass

Nonfood Sources

Body lotions
Lipstick
Medications and supplements

Pet food
Postage stamps and envelopes
Shampoo

milk and the various dairy products and how they help you stay strong and healthy. Let me articulate a framework around milk and why it should be taken out of your diet. Cow's milk is not a necessity for human health, unless you are a baby, and then you should be consuming breast milk from your mother! Humans are the only mammals that drink milk beyond their infancy, not to mention drink milk from another lactating species.

Gluten Cross-Reactivity

A host of health problems and autoimmune disorders have increasingly become associated with some of the most commonly consumed foods in the world, wheat and milk being the two most popular. Many of these problems can be traced to a concept termed molecular mimicry. The proteins found in such foods as milk and wheat are similar to those of human cells found in our nervous system and pancreas. This similarity can result in cross-reactivity that leads to food autoimmunity and even autoimmune disorders, such as multiple sclerosis, celiac disease, and neuromyelitis optica. Milk and the proteins found in dairy (casein, casomorphin, butyrophilin, and whey), oats, millet, soy, corn, and rice are common foods that possess the ability to mimic gluten and cause the same symptoms associated with nonceliac gluten sensitivity.

First, most of us are lactose intolerant, which is an impaired ability to digest lactose, a sugar found in milk and other dairy products. Lactose is normally broken down by an enzyme called lactase, which is produced by cells in the lining of the small intestine. Approximately 75 percent of the world's population has a reduced capacity or has completely lost the ability to digest lactose after infancy. Even if you could break down lactase, because it is a sugar, it quickly gets converted into glucose, which elevates blood sugar and thus inflammation. Inflammation is not your friend.

Next, if the gas and bloating from the lactose intolerance isn't enough to ditch the dairy, there is a protein in dairy known as casein that can cause problems. Casein can act like an excitotoxin, which can lead to neurodegenerative diseases. In addition, your immune system can confuse the casein molecule for gluten, especially for those with celiac disease or gluten intolerance (see above box). For those with an intolerance or sensitivity, it is critical to understand the concept of gluten cross-reactivity, or mimicry. Essentially, your body creates antibodies against gluten and can confuse those same antibodies as proteins found in other foods. When you eat those foods, even though they don't contain gluten, your body reacts as though they do. Even if you are completely gluten-free, you can still suffer all of the symptoms because your body thinks you are eating gluten.

Milk may also contain contaminants that range from hormones to pesticides. It naturally contains hormones and growth factors produced within a cow's body. But in addition, synthetic hormones, such as recombinant bovine growth hormone (rBGH), are commonly used in cows to increase the production of milk. Once introduced into the human body, these hormones may affect normal hormonal function, including insulin and estrogen. Also, when treating cows for such conditions as mastitis (inflammation of the mammary glands), antibiotics are used, and traces of these antibiotics have been found in samples of milk and dairy products. This treatment is used frequently, because mastitis is a common condition in cows, due to dairy product practices, which have cows producing more milk than nature intended. Pesticides, polychlorinated biphenyls (PCBs), and dioxins are other examples of contaminants found in milk.

Dairy products contribute one fourth to one half of the dietary intake of total dioxins. All of these toxins do not readily leave the body and can eventually build to harmful levels that may affect the immune, reproductive, and central nervous systems. Moreover, PCBs and dioxins have also been linked to cancer. It is estimated that each year 25 million pounds of antimicrobials are given to animals for nontherapeutic purpose and 1 million pounds are given for therapeutic purposes in contrast to the 3 million pounds ingested by humans. The potential health risks associated with growth hormones, antibiotics, and synthetic estrogens can cause decreased immunity, autoimmunity, neurologic damage, neuromusculoskeletal diseases, such as Parkinson's, and hormonal disruptions that can lead to infertility and thyroid disorders.

But what about my brittle bones? you ask. It is true that calcium is an important mineral that helps keep your bones strong. Our bones are constantly remodeling, meaning the body takes small amounts of calcium from the bones and replaces it with new calcium. But although calcium is necessary for optimal bone health, the actual benefits of calcium intake do not exist after consumption passes a certain threshold. Furthermore calcium works in conjunction with other vitamins and minerals, such as vitamins C, D, and K to create healthy bones. Clinical research shows that dairy products have little or no benefit for bones. The Harvard Nurses' Health Study, which followed more than seventy-two thousand women for eighteen years, showed no protective effect of increased milk consumption on fracture risk.

You can obtain all the calcium you need, without the dangers of food tolerances, cross-reactivity, or potential ingestion of hormones and antibiotics, by eating vegetables. You can decrease the risk of osteoporosis by reducing sodium intake in your diet, increasing your vegetable intake, and ensuring adequate calcium intake from plant foods, such as kale, broccoli, and other leafy green vegetables. Exercise, especially weight bearing and strength training, is also one of the most effective ways to increase bone density and decrease the risk of osteoporosis, and its benefits have been observed in studies of both children and adults. This is often the missing link in bone health.

What Contains Dairy?

More Obvious Sources of Dairy

Butter
Cheese
Cream
Cream-based sauces

Ice cream
Milk
Yogurt

Hidden Sources of Dairy

Au gratin foods
Bread, biscuits
Cakes, cookies
Candies
Chocolate
Chocolate drinks
Chowders
Crackers
Custards/pudding
Doughnuts
Flour mixes and batter
Gravy
Hot dogs

Mashed potatoes
Meat loaf
Omelets
Pancakes, waffles
Prescription and over-the-counter
    medications, including vitamin or
    other supplements, which often
    contain lactose
Salad dressings
Sauces
Soufflés
Soups

So Long, Sugar

Heather struggled with gluten intolerance for years. When she finally came to see me for headaches and balance issues, she was motivated and ready to try everything. Gluten and dairy were the first two things to go. She was thrilled not only that her headaches were 90 percent gone but also that she had lost 10 pounds in two weeks! With her headaches under control, her subsequent question was, "How do I lose the additional 10 pounds that is still hanging around?" Sugar was the next obvious place to look. But when I asked Heather about her sugar intake, she responded, "The only sugar I use is half a teaspoon of brown sugar in my tea in the morning." By the time we had dissected her diet and unearthed all the places that sugar hides, Heather was shocked by how much sugar had snuck into her diet. As mentioned earlier, all carbohydrates are broken down into sugar once digested. If you are eating foods with sugar added, no doubt your blood sugar is out of control and inflammation is rising.

The average American consumes approximately 150 pounds of sugar per year! Less than one hundred years ago, the average intake of sugar was only about 4 pounds per person per year. There is no doubt you have increased your consumption of sugar, and its health effects are taking a toll on your body. The primary sugars you encounter in your diet are sucrose and fructose. Fructose is a naturally occurring sugar found in fruit, where it serves as a marker for foods that are nutritionally rich. Historically, most Americans have consumed low quantities of fruit, one to two servings per day, which can be part of a healthy diet.

By far the most important sugar to eliminate is the modern, quite inflammatory and chemistry lab version of fructose: high-fructose corn syrup (HFCS), made from the overabundance of genetically modified corn. It has permeated our food supply. It is sweeter than either glucose or sucrose and serves to reward your taste buds with a sweet taste that provides a ton of calories but is completely void of much else in the way of nutrition. The intake of soft drinks containing HFCS or sucrose has risen in parallel with the obesity epidemic. A

2006 systematic review, covering almost twenty years of studies in the *American Journal of Clinical Nutrition*, found sufficient epidemiologic evidence indicating that a greater consumption of sugar-sweetened beverages is associated with weight gain and obesity. Soft drink consumption, which provides most of this form of fructose, has increased dramatically in the past six decades, rising from a per-person consumption of two servings per week in 1942 to that of two servings per day in 2000. High-fructose corn syrup is now used to sweeten tons of candies, juices, colas, cookies, cakes, and creams and has even found its way into less-tempting items, including bread, soups, snacks, and other packaged foods. Even your morning pumpkin spiced latte has high-fructose corn syrup in it!

High-fructose corn syrup works differently in the body than glucose. Both glucose and fructose are absorbed through the intestine, where they travel through the bloodstream. Glucose requires insulin to enter cells, such as muscle cells, to be stored for energy. Not only does this happen in muscle cells but it also occurs throughout various cells of the body. Insulin is the signal opening the door for your cells to store glucose for energy, so they can perform their essential functions. In comparison, fructose metabolism occurs primarily in the liver. When large amounts of fructose are ingested, as occurs in the case of HFCS, excessive production of triglycerides results, which can lead to insulin resistance, obesity, and inflammation. Numerous studies have even implicated HFCS as a potential risk factor for cardiovascular disease. A 2015 study in the *American Journal of Clinical Nutrition* found HFCS produced a significant increase in circulating blood lipids, a risk factor for cardiovascular disease and substantial evidence that the increasing consumption of added sugars is positively associated with cardiovascular disease. Furthermore, the researchers found a dose dependent relationship, meaning the more you consume, the worse it is for your health.

You have to be a sugar detective to figure out whether a packaged food contains added sugars, and you need to look carefully at the list of ingredients. Sugar has many other names. Besides those ending in "ose," such as maltose or sucrose, other names for sugar include high-fructose corn syrup, molasses, cane sugar, corn sweetener, raw sugar, syrup, agave, honey, or fruit juice concentrates. Just one 12-ounce can of regular soda contains eight teaspoons of sugar, or 130 calories and zero nutrition. It's time to eliminate all consumption of foods with high amounts of added sugars, such as sugar-sweetened beverages, once and for all.

Sugar is also highly addictive, especially high-fructose corn syrup. Shadowing the same receptor pathways of other addictive chemicals, including cocaine, HFCS alters the transmission of certain brain chemicals, including endorphins, dopamine, and serotonin, which in turn trigger the pleasure center of our brain, leaving us wanting more. A 2007 study found that intense sweetness surpasses cocaine reward even in addicted and drug-sensitized subjects. The alterations on brain function brought on by HFCS produce many of the hallmarks of addiction, including intense craving, the inability to control or stop use, a preoccupation with the food, and withdrawal symptoms. Sugar is addictive and should be eliminated as you recover and heal. Once you retrain your sweet tooth, you may find that you don't even miss so many of the foods you have been addicted to for so many years. And the best part is you will begin to enjoy other flavors food has to offer besides sweet.

The Many Names of Sugar

Agave nectar	Corn syrup	Fructose
Barley malt	Corn syrup solids	Fruit juice
Barbados sugar	Confectioners' sugar	Fruit juice concentrate
Beet sugar	Date sugar	Galactose
Brown sugar	Dehydrated cane juice	Glucose
Buttered syrup	Demerara sugar	Glucose solids
Cane juice	Dextran	Golden sugar
Cane sugar	Dextrose	Golden syrup
Caramel	Diastatic malt	Grape sugar
Carob syrup	Diatase	High-fructose corn syrup
Castor sugar	Ethyl maltol	Icing sugar

continues

The Many Names of Sugar   *continued*

Invert sugar	Molasses	Sorghum syrup
Lactose	Monk fruit	Sucrose
Malt	Panocha	Sugar (granulated)
Maltodextrin	Powdered sugar	Treacle
Maltose	Raw sugar	Turbinado sugar
Malt syrup	Refiners' syrup	Yellow sugar
Mannitol	Rice syrup	
Maple syrup	Sorbitol	

Say No to GMOs

GMOs are a new area of science that promote the promise of helping to alleviate global food shortages and product shelf life, improvements in livestock, and breeding crop yields that are insect, pest, disease, and weather resistant, but they also hold hidden dangers. Genetically modified foods have had their DNA altered through genetic engineering in a laboratory. The United States is the world's leader in the production of GMO crops, and currently the FDA does not require foods that have been genetically modified to be labeled as such. The state of Vermont has been the most successful and aggressive with GMO legislation; other states have faced significant pushback from lobbyists and special-interest groups. The most commonly grown GMOs are corn, soybeans, cotton, sugar beets, and canola. In more than sixty countries around the world, including Australia, Japan, and all of the countries in the European Union, there are significant restrictions or complete bans on the production and sale of GMOs, and many countries require them to be labeled. In the United States, the government has approved GMOs based on studies conducted by the same corporations that created them and profit from their sale—an inherent conflict of interest. Labeling of genetically modified foods is not required in the United States, despite the clear desire of the public to have as much information as possible about their food. There is very little epidemiological research on the long-term effects of GMOs on the environment, our food supply, or our health.

More Americans are taking matters into their own hands and purchasing only non-GMO foods when possible. It would be wonderful
if we knew exactly how these plants and foods affected not only our
body but also the larger ecosystem and globe, but we just don't have
the studies. Until then I believe we should all—including our government and large food manufacturers—proceed with caution when it
comes to GMOs. When the health of humans and the environment is
at stake, it may not be necessary to wait for scientific certainty to take
protective action.

GMOs and Glyphosate

More concerning is the case that GMO crops are herbicide-resistant
crops. Herbicide resistance is the ability of a plant to survive and re-
produce, following the application and exposure to a dose of herbicide. GMOs are bred to be genetically resistant to herbicides. As more
GMO plants are developed, glyphosate use is on the rise. Glyphosate, commonly known as Roundup, is an herbicide used to kill weeds.
GMO plants are bred to tolerate glyphosate and its use. The more
glyphosate is used on crops, the more exposure we have as humans by
ingesting it directly via food and indirectly in our water supply.

The companies that produce glyphosate claim that the herbicide
and GMO crops are safe. However, a study in the journal *Reproductive Toxicology* found that the herbicides used on genetically modified
(GM) crops and, in some cases, the genes used to create GM crops, are
able to survive in our digestive tract and move into our bloodstream.
They even found them to be able to cross the placenta of the developing fetus of women who were pregnant. Use of herbicides has also led
to groundwater contaminations, the death of several wildlife species,
and has been attributed to various human and animal illnesses. As glyphosate use is on the rise in developing countries, farmers are coming
into closer contact with the chemical and experiencing adverse health
effects, toxicity, and even death. One study found cardiac arrhythmias
in people who came in contact with glyphosate.

Glyphosate is also commonly used for desiccation and ripening
right before the harvest. This farming practice ensures that glyphosate

residues are present in our food supply. A 2013 study in the *Journal of Toxicology* discussed how the rise of celiac disease and gluten intolerance is caused by the use of glyphosate and concluded with a plea to governments to reconsider policies regarding the safety of glyphosate residues in foods.

Eliminating GMOs are crucial for healing your leaky gut, because the major problem with GMOs is that they can do damage to your digestive tract and *cause* a leaky gut. Genetically modified corn has been engineered to produce its own insecticide called BT-toxin, which is produced in every cell of the plant. This toxin works to kill insects by creating holes in their digestive tract. And you're eating it when you eat GMO products. GMOs can disrupt the lining of your gut, triggering leaky gut and the sequel of pain syndromes.

Glyphosate's disruption of the body's ability to detoxify environmental toxins leads to enhanced toxicity, thereby increasing the damaging effects of other food-borne chemical residues and environmental toxins. Although the impact on the body is not immediate, it insidiously manifests slowly over time as inflammation and damages cellular systems throughout the body. Consequences are most of the diseases and conditions associated with a Western diet, which include gastrointestinal disorders, obesity, diabetes, heart disease, depression, autism, infertility, cancer, and Alzheimer's disease. Glyphosate also destroys the healthy microbiome that lives in your intestines, and this disruption has been linked to obesity. In fact, the obesity epidemic began in the United States in the 1970s, just as glyphosate was being used on crops and introduced into the food chain. As its use has steadily increased in agriculture so have our country's obesity rates.

Not Soy Fast

Genetically modified soy was introduced to the United States in 1996, and these soybeans now account for almost 90 percent of all soy produced and consumed. Soy is another ingredient that has become persistent throughout our food supply. As people have become aware that we should avoid dairy milk, we have substituted it with the equally problematic soy milk. And we have not stopped here, as soy is used to make fake cheese and meat products. In many circles, soy is touted as a health food. There is even soy ice cream! Soy-based products and tofu are used almost exclusively in many vegan and Asian dishes. Soybean oil are also frequently used in the frying of foods, margarines, and butter substitutes. If you can't believe it's not butter, it's probably soybean oil! Soy is also found in cosmetics, hand sanitizer, lotion, shampoo, conditioner, soap, medications, vitamins, and supplements.

One way to develop food intolerances is to be bombarded with them every day. GMO products, due to their availability, are now used in thousands of foods, which means you are exposed to them regularly and are building up an intolerance. Contrary to popular advertising, soy isn't a miracle health food. It has been implicated in a number of health problems, including thyroid dysfunction, reproductive disorders, cognitive decline, digestive problems, and decreased sperm counts. It is relatively new to our food supply (less than one thousand years old), and because of this, it has a higher rate of potential allergenicity and intolerance.

Soy also contains phytates, which can bind to minerals and lead to nutrient deficiencies. Soybeans are high in phytic acid, present in the bran or hulls of all seeds. It's a substance that can block the uptake of essential minerals, such as calcium, magnesium, copper, iron, and especially zinc, in the intestinal tract. Soy's effects on the thyroid involve the critical relationship between iodine status and thyroid function, including iodine deficiency. The wide consumption of soy products may cause weight gain by either estrogenic or goitrogenic (thyroid-inhibiting) activity, thus causing hypothyroidism and the development of increased visceral and adipose fat.

What Contains Soy?

More Obvious Sources of Soy

Edamame	Nimame	Soy flour
Hydrolyzed soy protein	Soy albumin	Soy grits
Miso	Soy beer	Soy ice cream
Natto	Soy cheese	Soy meal

continues

What Contains Soy? *continued*		
Soy milk	Soy sauce	Soybeans
Soy nuts	Soy sprouts	Soybean oil
Soy pasta	Soy yogurt	Tofu
Soy protein	Soya	Yuba
Hidden Sources of Soy		
Kinako	Shoyu	Teriyaki sauce
Mono-/diglycerides	Tamari	Textured vegetable
MSG	Tempeh	protein

Kick the Corn Habit

Seen by most as a vegetable, corn is actually a grain and the most popular crop grown in the United States. The corn you currently eat, with its bright yellow color and sweet taste, is far from the original corn Native Americans consumed centuries ago. Corn has been hybridized and genetically modified to taste sweeter and is now ubiquitous in our food supply. Corn oil, corn syrup, high-fructose corn syrup, and cornstarch can be found in most processed food. Corn has a large abundance of omega-6 fatty acids, with a ratio of 46:1. Remember, you want your ratio of omega-6 to omega-3 to be a minimum of 4:1 but preferably leaning toward 1:1. Corn, along with soy, is the primary grain fed to farm animals and livestock to fatten them up. When livestock is fed a diet of corn, the omega-6 to omega-3 ratio is changed, so the meat you are eating is less nutritious. Avoid feeding yourself as if you were livestock.

We have known the effects of corn on pain for decades. A 1981 study in the *British Medical Journal* reported the case of a woman whose battle with rheumatoid arthritis suddenly ended when it was discovered that her symptoms were triggered by corn products. Corn was eliminated from her diet and, after twenty-five years of joint pains, her symptoms completely disappeared. Six weeks later the patient began to develop joint pain once again. It was discovered that the cook preparing her food had started using cornstarch as a thickening agent. After eliminating the cornstarch, her symptoms vanished yet again. In 1991, researchers in Oslo, Norway, reported in the *Lancet* a study in which they eliminated foods believed to be common arthritis triggers in a group of twenty-six arthritis patients. Corn was one of the foods eliminated. The average pain score fell from over 5, on a scale from 0 to 10, to under 3. Joint stiffness, swelling, and tenderness diminished, and grip strength also improved. Most important, the benefits were sustained on reexamination a year later.

Now that you know corn is a grain, it's also important to realize that it is very starchy and has a high glycemic index. That means that most of the corn you are eating is converted into sugar, causing a spike in insulin. This is not the "vegetable" you want to fill your plate with. There is a good reason it is called sweet corn and why you have an addiction to popcorn and can't stop eating it.

The Many Names of Corn

Aspartame (artificial sweetener)	Cellulose microcrystalline
Astaxanthin	Choline chloride
Baking powder	Citric acid
Bleached flour	Citrus cloud emulsion (CCS)
Blended sugar (sugaridextrose)	Confectioners' sugar
Calcium citrate	Corn
Calcium fumarate	Corn alcohol
Calcium gluconate	Corn extract
Calcium lactate	Corn flour
Calcium magnesium acetate (CMA)	Corn gluten
	Cornmeal
Calcium stearate	Corn oil, corn oil margarine
Calcium stearoyl lactylate	Cornstarch (a.k.a. cornflour)
Caramel and caramel color	Corn sweetener, corn sugar
Carboxymethylcellulose sodium	Corn syrup, corn syrup solids
Cellulose, methyl	Crosscarmellose sodium
Cellulose, powdered	Crystalline dextrose
Cetearyl glucoside	Crystalline fructose

continues

The Many Names of Corn   *continued*

Cyclodextrin
DATUM (a dough conditioner)
Decyl glucoside
Decyl polyglucose
Dextrin
Dextrose (also found in
    IV solutions)
D-gluconic acid
Distilled white vinegar
Drying agent
Erythorbic acid
Erythritol
Ethanol
Ethocel 20
Ethylcellulose
Ethylene
Ethyl acetate
Ethyl alcohol
Ethyl lactate
Ethyl maltol
Fibersol-2
Flavorings
Food starch
Fructose
Fruit juice concentrate
Fumaric acid
Germ/germ meal
Gluconate
Gluconic acid
Glucono delta-lactone
Gluconolactone
Glucosamine
Glucose
Glucose syrup (also found in
    IV solutions)
Glutamate
Gluten

Gluten feed/meal
Glycerides
Glycerin
Glycerol
Golden syrup
Grits
High-fructose corn syrup
Horniny
Honey
Hydrolyzed corn
Hydrolyzed corn protein
Hydrolyzed vegetable protein
Hydroxypropyl methylcellulose
Lauryl glucoside
Magnesium citrate
Magnesium fumarate
Magnesium stearate
Maize
Malt syrup from corn
Malt, malt extract
Maltitol
Maltodextrin
Maltol
Maltose
Mannitol
Methyl gluceth
Methyl glucose
Methyl glucoside
Methylcellulose
Microcrystaline cellulose
Modified cellulose gum
Modified cornstarch
Molasses (corn syrup may be present; know
    your product)
Mono-/diglycerides
MSG (monosodium glutamate)
Natural flavorings

continues

The Many Names of Corn   *continued*

Olestra/Olean
Polenta
Polydextrose
Polylactic acid (PLA)
Polysorbates
Polyvinyl acetate
Potassium citrate
Potassium fumarate
Potassium gluconate
Powdered sugar
Pregelatinized starch
Propionic acid
Propylene glycol
Propylene glycol monostearate
Semolina (unless from wheat)
Simethicone
Sodium citrate
Sodium erythorbate
Sodium fumarate
Sodium lactate
Sodium starch glycolate
Sodium stearoyl fumarate

Sorbate
Sorbic acid
Sorbitan (anything)
Sorbitol
Sorghum (not all is bad; the syrup and/or
    grain can be mixed with corn)
Splenda (artificial sweetener)
Starch
Stearic acid
Stearoyls
Sucralose
Sucrose
Treacle (a.k.a. golden syrup)
Triethyl citrate
Unmodified starch
Vanilla, natural flavoring
Vanilla, pure or extract
Vanillin
Vinyl acetate
Yeast
Zea mays
Zein

Lurking in the Shadows: Nightshades

Colorful bell peppers, tomatoes, potatoes, and eggplants have a variety of phytonutrients that are beneficial for your health. These are not high on the list of foods that
cause pain, due to their nutrient content and health-promoting antioxidants. Unfortunately, however, for many patients with a leaky gut, autoimmune disease, or osteoarthritis, the nightshade family of vegetables can be problematic. The nightshades
contain glycoalkyloids, which are known to cause a leaky gut. Tobacco, also a nightshade plant, should not be a part of your life—in any form! Numerous studies have
linked cigarette smoking to painful syndromes, not to mention it is a proven carcino-
gen. Many people find relief by minimizing the amount of nightshades, such as tomatoes and peppers, or by eliminating them from their diet. However, most will find that
once you follow the 4R protocol and heal your leaky gut, you will be able to tolerate
nightshade family of vegetables without a problem.

Eggs, Not Always So Excellent

If you have a healthy gut and don't struggle with pain, eggs are in some ways a perfect food. But they're not a perfect idea for *everyone* and not all the time, because they can be a major trigger for persistent leaky gut as well as joint pain. Our hunter-gatherer ancestors were opportunists. They would consume eggs whenever they were available, but they wouldn't consume them every day, day in and day out, for the entire year. That's the pattern that we see today: dietary monotony, where people eat the same foods every day. If you don't have an allergy or autoimmune diseases, eat as many eggs as you like, because the cholesterol issue is a nonissue. During the gut healing phase, though, you will refrain from eating eggs to make sure that they are not causing any type of leaky gut or exacerbating your pain in any way.

The type of egg you purchase is important as well. Conventional factory eggs are laid by hens that have spent the majority of their lives "cooped up" in warehouse-size buildings, without access to the outdoor environment. They are fed a diet primarily of GMO (genetically modified) corn and soy, laden with antibiotics and hormones. These have the potential to wind up in the egg. When purchasing eggs, you should opt for USDA organic omega-3-enriched eggs. These are from hens that have been fed an omega-3-enriched feed from flax- and chia seeds and are allowed to roam freely eating grass and bugs, their native diet. Organic hens lay eggs that are higher in vitamins A and E, and omega-3s. A study compared the fatty acid composition of three types of eggs: conventional, organic, and omega-3-enriched. Omega-3-enriched eggs had 39 percent less arachidonic acid, an inflammatory omega-6 fatty acid that most people consume too much. Omega-3-enriched eggs had five times as much omega-3 as the conventional eggs.

Eggs are also one of the most common foods people are allergic to, and people often also have food sensitivities to them. Egg intolerance develops when the body's immune system becomes sensitized and overreacts to protein in the egg white. When eggs are eaten, the body sees the protein as a foreign invader and sends out chemicals to attack. Those chemicals cause the symptoms of an allergic reaction. Most people who are allergic to hen's eggs have antibodies that react to one of four proteins in the egg white: ovomucoid, ovalbumin, ovotransferrin, and lysozyme. Lysozyme is perhaps the largest culprit in the egg. This enzyme found in the egg white is designed to protect the egg yolk from foreign invaders, such as bacteria. Lysosyme does an excellent job at gobbling up bacteria so it does not reach the yolk, but the challenge is it easily passes through your digestive system and gut lining. Indirectly, the lysozyme and the bacteria it swallowed can be nicely transported and circulated around your body. The egg yolk contains several potential triggers as well, although overall the egg white is the most problematic. A person may react only to a protein in the egg white and may be able to easily tolerate yolk. Some people will be allergic to proteins in both the egg white and the egg yolk. The yolk is the part of the egg that contains DHA and EPA fatty acids (if they are from pasture-raised chickens!).

Be Wary of "Chicken Shots"

Suzanne struggled with knee pain for almost six months and was determined not to have surgery or go on medication. She already had a history of an ulcer due to a prescribed anti-inflammatory drug. She spoke with her doctor, did her own research, and opted for an injection that promised to help lubricate her knee and provide cushioning for the joint and offer up to six months of pain relief for her osteoarthritic knee. To her surprise, it caused severe pain, swelling, and localized redness. She could barely walk and had to resort to powerful pain meds to get through the first week. Eventually, she had to have her knee aspirated (fluid taken out with a needle) due to the amount of swelling. The viscosupplement in the injection she received was made from chicken combs. Use caution when having one of these injections in case you are allergic to avian proteins, feathers, and egg products. A trial of eliminating eggs from your diet to lower inflammation is a much easier and safer way than injecting proteins into your knee that could cause an allergic reaction and worsen your joint pain.

Hidden Eggs		
Breads	French toast	Mayonnaise
Breaded foods	Fritters	Meat loaf
Cakes	Frostings	Meringues
Cookies	Frying batter	Pancakes, waffles
Cream	Hollandaise sauce	Salad dressings
Cream sauces	Ice cream	Sausages
Egg noodles	Macaroons	Sherbets
Flour mixes	Marshmallows	Soufflés

Purge Your Pantry

Foods you desire most tend to cause the most problems—you crave them because you are addicted to them. A huge part of your success will begin with your preparedness. Some of the foods discussed have been a staple in your life. You even may have looked at them as health foods! Now that you understand how even such foods as granola and whole-grain bread can be harming your health instead of helping you recover, you not only need to keep them off your plate but also keep them out of your pantry. Willpower is for the weak. The strong ones know exactly what their poison is and avoid it at all costs. Many of these foods you have been addicted to for years, and having them around is dangerous for your health.

If you are like most of my clients, you may store food like a chipmunk. Begin with your kitchen, including all cupboards, your refrigerator, and the pantry. Read all labels on all boxes and packages for any of the five foods and where they may be hiding. Place them all in a bag and bring them to the nearest food pantry or your local place of worship. Foods tend to linger in certain places as well. Our big-box supermarkets have turned our homes into food warehouses. Check your basement, garage, outdoor kitchen, or any other place you may have foods stashed away. Make a list of the five foods to avoid, and pin it on your refrigerator and tape it to the back of your cell phone case as a reminder. Also make sure to check your car. At work, check your desk and the company kitchen. If you share a kitchen with co-workers, tell them that you have a recent food allergy and will need to modify your diet until you heal. In three weeks they will be eager to know exactly what you are doing as your waist shrinks, energy increases, and vitality returns.

Tips for Dining Out

- View the menu online ahead of time.
- Be the one to choose the restaurant when going out with friends, to ensure that it has healthy options you can eat.
- Call ahead. Call before dining and let the restaurant staff know that you avoid certain foods.
- Avoid bakeries: There is a high risk of cross-contamination, since many items are made with some of the top foods you need to avoid, such as egg, gluten, dairy, corn, sugar, and soy.
- Exercise extreme caution with restaurants that serve premade foods. The staff may not have an accurate list of the ingredients in a premade item.
- Avoid restaurants that are known to use allergens in many dishes. For instance, Asian cuisines often use soy in their recipes.

Adding Probiotic Foods/Fermented Foods

As you begin to take away food that has been causing you pain and making you fat, your microbiome will begin to change. A shift in the type and quantity of bacteria in your gut will help it to rebalance in the favorable direction of health and healing. Many of the foods you have been eating up until now promote small intestinal bacterial overgrowth (SIBO) and have been a major contributor to your symptoms and weight gain. Think about your lawn when it begins to regrow from a long winter's freeze. The lawn is mostly brown and what little grass is attempting to grow is competing with weeds. It's important to bolster your system with probiotic and fermented foods, as we mentioned earlier in the chapter during the 4R Gut-Healing Program.

If fermented foods are completely new to your system, you may experience mild to moderate symptoms, which are completely natural and healthy for your body. These symptoms can include gas, breakouts, headaches, and more. Just note that you have to give your body time to adjust and adapt. None of this is bad; in fact, only good things are happening. Your body is getting rid of toxins that need to be released. This is important, because the fermented foods are replacing those toxins with beneficial, life-enhancing organisms that will ultimately make you feel and look great!

If fermented foods are not palatable, you can take a probiotic supplement in their place. Probiotics supplements are a powerful way to reinoculate your gut with healthy bacteria. The two most common strains studied are lactobacillus and bifidobacterium. Choose a supplement that has a diversity of strains of each, as this will help to balance your microbiome. Both have been shown to improve the intestinal barrier function by increasing tight junctions and reducing inflammation. Along with eliminating the five foods, these two probiotics have been shown to help even the worst intestinal diseases, such as ulcerative colitis. As with any probiotic, start with a lower dose and progressively work your way up over a period of one to two weeks. Small doses can be taken by breaking a capsule and placing it in your food or drink. Probiotics should first be taken with food but over time, as your microbiome improves, you can take them with water between meals for maximum efficiency.

4R Gut-Healing Nutrient Protocols

The 4R program can lead to dramatic improvement in your symptoms through avoiding certain foods and adding others. However, healing a leaky gut also requires some help to reestablish a healthy microbiome, decrease inflammation, and repair your gut, so you may need to add supplements to your daily regimen. The following table provides nutrient support for healing a leaky gut. A comprehensive table is also available for you in Appendix B. For more on gut-healing supplement protocols, visit www.drjoetatta.com/guthealing.

Getting Started: A 7-Day Gut-Healing Meal Plan

This is not a hunger strike, and if you follow my suggested meal plans, you will have platefuls of nutritious healthy food. Planning and

4R Gut-Healing Program

Supplement	Dosage	Notes
Remove Botanical for treating SIBO	1 capsule daily	Botanical blend including extracts from berbine (*Berberis vulgaris*), oregano (*Origanum vulgare*), grapefruit (*Citrus paradisi*).
Replace Digestive enzyme	1 capsule with meals	Enzyme blend including betaine HCl, amylase, protease, pepsin, lactase, and lipase.
Repopulate Probiotics	1–2 capsules daily	50–100 billion IU per capsule blend of live cultures containing lactobacillis and bifidobacterium strains. Avoid probiotics that are not gluten-, soy-, corn-, and dairy-free.
Repair L-glutamine	1–2 g 2x/day	An essential amino acid needed by the body for repair of the digestive tract and enterocytes in the gut. L-L-Glutamate, in addition to fiber, serves as a fuel precursor for colonocytes.
Gut formula	Once daily	Gut repair formulas include a combination of vitamins, minerals, and herbs including: deglycyrrhizinated licorice, aloe vera extract, slippery elm, marshmallow, MSM, chamomile, mucin, okra extract, quercetin, zinc, N-acetyl glucosamine, vitamin D.

preparing is the best way to achieve success. First, visit www.drjoe tatta.com/shoppingguide and download your free shopping guide and food list. Take this to the grocery store with you when you shop and use it as a resource when you are looking at food items. Having this will greatly improve your chance of success. Next, make sure to read all food labels and become familiar with the lists of where each of the five foods to eliminate hides. I've included additional recipes in Appendix A at the back of the book.

Meal Timing

Begin your day with a healing protein shake.

Your first meal should be within an hour of getting out of bed.

Meals should be spread out every four to six hours and you should only eat three meals a day.

	Sunday	Monday	Tuesday	Wednesday	Thursday	Friday	Saturday
Breakfast	Strawberry Vanilla Shake	Chocolate Avocado Shake	Mint Chip Shake	Chocolate Cherry Shake	Mexican Chocolate Shake	Vanilla Almond Espresso Shake	Green Tea Protein Shake
Lunch	Kale Sausage Bean Soup	Roasted Chicken and Vegetables	Colorful Quinoa and Black Bean Casserole	Dr. Joe's Favorite Salad topped with pomegranate seeds and walnuts	Turkey Patties Roasted Beet and Orange Salad	Colorful Quinoa and Black Bean Casserole	Lentil Veggie Sauté
Dinner	Roasted Chicken and Vegetables	Slow Cooker Beef Brisket	Rosemary Garlic Lamb Chops Roasted Beet and Orange Salad	Grilled Chicken with 50/50 Mixed Green Salad with Grilled Salmon	Chicken Breast with Persimmon Salsa Baked Acorn Squash	Quinoa Pasta with Meatballs Eggplant Medley	Baked Salmon with Chives

Stay Hydrated

Your body will also begin to detoxify itself, clearing metabolites and waste products through urinating, defecating, sweating, and breathing. It is essential that you stay hydrated to help flush toxins out of your system. It's important to drink water daily, because dehydration is a major contributor to pain and stiffness. I recommend a minimum of six glasses of water per day. You will also be getting more water into your diet by consuming healthy vegetables, which have a high concentration of water. Herbal teas in their many flavors are also allowed,

Popular Food Substitutions

The following are a few suggestions for ways to replace some of your favorite foods that you have now eliminated from your diet.

Sugar: organic stevia

Milk and yogurt: almond, coconut, hemp, hazelnut, oat, or rice milk and coconut yogurt (Read the labels to make sure there are not additives or sweeteners and that the oat milk is gluten-free. Always choose the unsweetened versions, to avoid extra calories and sugar.)

Butter and margarine: olive or coconut oil, coconut oil spread, ghee (clarified butter)

Bread, chips, crackers: gluten-free breads, chips, and crackers made with chia, flax, quinoa, amaranth

Pasta: quinoa pasta, spaghetti squash, zucchini noodles, or gluten-free pastas made from a combination of brown rice, quinoa, and amaranth (not corn- or soy-based pasta!)

Parmesan cheese: nutritional yeast

Condiments: salt, pepper, basil, oregano, marjoram, rosemary, sage, carob, cinnamon, parsley, tarragon, thyme, turmeric (avoid all hot/spicy peppers)

Soy sauce: coconut aminos

Flour and baking: gluten-free vegan flour mixes, almond flour, coconut flour, sweet potato flour, plantain flour

Drinks: sparkling or mineral water; natural flavor-enhanced water made with lemon, lime, strawberries, mint, or unsweetened coconut water; caffeine-free organic teas

and green tea is preferred in this phase of the diet. Don't have more than one cup per day or any caffeine past two p.m. Coffee (regular and decaf) is not allowed in this phase of the diet. While not high on the list of foods people are sensitive to, coffee can cause both blood sugar and stress hormones to rise, which means belly fat storage begins. If you are a caffeine junkie, I recommend weaning your intake down over the course of a week to eliminate the symptoms of caffeine withdrawal, which may include headaches, fatigue, fogginess, and irritability. Once you are off the morning mud, you will see how nutrient-dense food will provide all the energy you need. Obviously, artificially sweetened and regular soft drinks are not in any part of the Healing Pain Program. You may have seltzer or still water mixed with lemon or lime, or infused with mint or berries. These make great beverages to begin digestion in the morning.

After 21 Days: Reintroducing Foods

Within four to seven days, many people begin to notice the remarkable effects of the Healing Pain Program, with less joint pain, muscle aches, and headaches; increased energy; and less abdominal pain and irritable bowel symptoms. Trust me, once you ditch the dairy, go gluten-free, and figure out some of your other food sensitivities, you will instantly see how much better you feel. After twenty-one days, you may find that certain foods still cause you to have throngs of pain, stiffness, and weight gain. This means you have an intolerance to those foods, and it would be best to continue to avoid them indefinitely. Personally, gluten *never* agrees with me, so I have eliminated it from my diet completely! Some people feel so much better on this phase of the Healing Pain Diet Program that they choose to remain off certain foods forever, 100 percent of the time. If you are one of these people, congratulations, as you are one of the select few who really listens to your "gut" and reaps the rewards of living healthy each day. If you struggle with a chronic inflammation, pain, or autoimmune condition, even once your gut is fully healed, you may have to avoid certain foods 90 percent of the time or more.

By now you should understand that added sugar has no room in your diet 95 percent of the time, so we do not need to test or reintroduce it. And corn, used to make high-fructose corn syrup, which is more sugar, is gone as well. If you can find 100 percent organic non-GMO corn on the cob (or in any other form), you can have that once a week, but you probably need to find a very old Incan or Native American strain. Since most of you are not shopping for food on a reservation, it's highly unlikely you will find this type of corn. That leaves us with just four foods to test (gluten, dairy, eggs, and soy).

After twenty-one days, you may choose to reintroduce foods back into your diet, one at a time, and see how you respond. Here is a quick guide on how to get started on the reintroduction (more detailed information and support can be found at www.drjoetatta.com /reintroduction):

1. Reintroduce only one new food at a time. Make sure not to reintroduce any of the other foods! Introducing one food at a time helps identify whether that particular food is causing an issue. If you introduce more than one, you won't know which food is the problem.

2. On a Monday and Tuesday, reintroduce gluten into your diet, as this is often one of the most problematic foods. Eat it twice a day and then stop eating it and wait 48 hours to see whether you have a reaction. This is easiest by eating products that contain wheat. For example, eat some type of gluten twice on Monday and on Tuesday, such as a cup of whole wheat pasta or a sandwich with whole wheat bread.

3. If you are extremely sensitive or intolerant to certain foods, you may notice symptoms immediately. Stop eating this food immediately if symptoms develop.

4. If you don't have a reaction to the food immediately, continue to watch for symptoms on Wednesday and Thursday, as they may be delayed. This does not necessarily mean that symptoms, such as pain, will be less severe; it just means there can be a lag time as your immune system is ramping up inflammation. For some it may take up to four days to notice a reaction.

5. Assess your response over the four-day period, keeping track of your symptoms (a list of common reactions follows). If there is no reaction to a food, you can keep that food in your food plan and continue with the next food for reintroduction. If you are unsure whether you had a reaction, retest the same food in the same manner.

6. Follow the same routine as above with dairy next, then eggs, and finally soy.

Common Reactions include
- Aches and pains: muscles, joints, tendons, or ligaments
- Headaches or dizziness
- Any gastrointestinal symptoms, such as stomach pain, heartburn, nausea, constipation, diarrhea, gas, bloating, undigested/partially digested food particles in stool
- Fatigue or low energy
- Strong food cravings: sugar cravings, fat cravings, pica (mineral cravings)
- Trouble either falling asleep or staying asleep or not feeling as rested
- Skin rashes, acne, dry skin, bumps or spots
- Mood issues: feeling depressed, anxious, or stressed

Food Reintroduction Calendar

	Day 1	Day 2	Day 3	Day 4
Digestive problems				
Joint/muscle pain				
Headaches				
Skin problems				
Sleep disturbances				
Energy level				
Brain fog				

Gut-Healing Shopping List

You can follow the same shopping list on page 96 in Chapter 5, but here are a few specific ideas for items that may help when you are eliminating foods.

Nongluten Grains and Flours

Amaranth	Quinoa
Arrowroot flour	Rice
Buckwheat	Sorghum
Coconut flour	Tapioca
Garbanzo (chickpea) flour	Teff
Millet	Wild rice
Nut flours	
Oats (must be certified gluten free!)	

Dairy Substitutions

Almond milk	Coconut yogurt (to replace
Cashew milk	dairy or soy yogurt)
Coconut butter	Ghee (in place of butter)
Coconut milk	Hemp milk

Hopefully, now that you have eliminated the top five gut-damaging foods from your diet, you are feeling a noticeable difference in all areas of your body, including those joints that give you the most trouble or pain. You've likely also lost at least 10 pounds by this point, which is having a direct effect on your overall pain scale. But you may still be struggling, unable to shed the pain or the pounds. If that's the case, take a careful look at Chapter 7, where we'll cover a more intense program to help your body get back on track. To learn more about healing your gut, visit www.drjoetatta.com/guthealth.

Dr. Joe's Pain Relief Reminders

- A leaky gut, when toxic material passes through the walls of the digestive tract, can create inflammation and therefore persistent pain.
- Your 4R gut-healing protocol comprises Remove, Replace, Repopulate, and Repair.
- The five foods to eliminate pain are: gluten, dairy, sugar, eggs, and GMOs (especially corn and soy). Remember that they often hide in unexpected or tricky places!
- Eliminate the five foods for at least three weeks and consider weaning them out of your diet indefinitely.
- Add supportive supplements, such as a probiotic, digestive enzyme, and gut-healing formula to assist with healing.

7

KETOGENIC HEALING

The Basics of Ketogenic Healing

Time frame: Three weeks.

Changes: Significantly increase the amount of healthy fat and decrease the amount of carbohydrates to shift the body from utilizing glucose as its primary fuel to using ketone bodies. Continue to eliminate the five foods discussed in Chapter 6, although eggs are allowed here if tolerated, due to their utilization as a ketogenic food.

Supportive supplementation: Follow the 4R gut-healing supplement protocol.

Results: Those with resistant weight loss and the most persistent pain often see the most dramatic improvements cycling to a ketogenic diet for three weeks, with 10 pounds of weight loss and almost complete resolution of pain.

You may still be struggling. Persistent pain, low energy, and extra weight are still a significant problem. You are feeling hopeless, helpless, and discouraged. If you are anything like me, you always want to peel back one more layer of the onion to see whether you get any closer to the root of the problem. There is always a path toward healing—it just may not be the same path that worked for your friend or cousin. Remember, each of us is biochemically unique and what works for one may not work for another. Your chemistry is unique to your genetics, habits, and environment. You may have been in a state of metabolic mayhem for longer than others, and you need more help. Instead of continuing to damage your metabolism, let's recommit to resuming the healing journey together. I'm in this with you and understand how tough it can be, especially when you are living with pain.

After completing the gut-healing phase, you may very well be happy with the amount of weight you have lost and how much pain has been alleviated. However, if you still have weight-loss goals and pain persists, I suggest you progress through to ketogenic healing. This may benefit you if:

- You have difficulty losing weight.
- You gain weight easily.
- You can easily correlate pain with eating.
- You think you have a slow metabolism.

It will also help if you struggle with the following issues and symptoms, even after you've eliminated the five foods during gut healing in the previous chapter:

- Fatigue
- Brain fog
- Persistent pain
- Migraines
- A neurodegenerative disease (e.g., Parkinson's)
- Autoimmune problems (e.g., rheumatoid arthritis, lupus)
- Prediabetes or type 2 diabetes
- Insulin resistance
- Metabolic syndrome
- Nonalcoholic fatty liver disease (NAFLD)
- Obesity

The low-carbohydrate and ketogenic approach is a rapid and personalized way for you to alleviate the chronic disease that is causing your pain. Food is your medicine and your entry point for healing. Always remember that the foods you eat, along with the lifestyle you lead, can reverse chronic inflammation and your disease. The Healing Pain Program is a revolutionary plan designed to empower you on your path to health and recovery. The future of medicine has arrived where healing is in your hands and customized to your unique chemistry and life. Learning which diet is best for you and having the faith to try different approaches allows food to be part of a medicinal approach to health and healing. Gut healing and ketogenic healing provide you with two paths to recovering your health. Once you have met your health goals, you may transition back to gut healing or the core nutritional healing plan, as long as you can maintain a healthy body composition and pain does not return.

Flipping the Fat-Loss Switch in Your Cells

If you have had a difficult time losing weight or keeping the weight off, you are not alone. More than 80 percent of people who begin a diet regain weight within two years of losing it. Typically, this is because the diet they chose was one that simply reduced calories drastically. I want you to *stop* dieting and *start* learning what it takes to steer yourself toward real recovery. I want you to understand how your body and cells work, so that you know your options. In the previous chapter, you learned how to heal your gut and lower inflammation naturally. In this section, you will learn how to shift from a state of resistant weight loss to becoming an all-day fat burner.

Mitomaximize Your Health

For years, we placed emphasis on calories and not enough on nutrition. Reducing calories is pointless if you only eat unhealthy processed food. What you place on your dinner plate will either serve to harm or help your recovery. If there is one tenet I want you to walk away with from this book, it is that getting proper nutrition into your body is the first and fastest way to end pain and lead an active life. The food you eat gets broken down and dictates how your body functions. If you are eating a poor diet, you may be unknowingly turning on certain genes that make you susceptible to certain diseases. Conversely, if you are eating nutrient-dense foods, they not only prevent disease but also help you recover from the pain and disability that many chronic diseases carry.

For example, I recently purchased a gas-powered lawn mower. When I returned home, I filled it with some gasoline, pulled the starter rope, and expected it to start moving. The engine made some noise, ran for a few moments, and then petered out with a puff of black smoke. When I read the directions more carefully, I realized that this type of lawn mower required a special oil that is actually a combination of oil and gas. For every gallon of gas, I had to mix in 2 ounces of oil for the lawn mower to work properly. Your body is similar—you need the right blend of nutrients to feed your cells, otherwise they do not function properly. Nowhere is this more important than deep inside your cells where energy is made.

If you are not feeding your cells the nutrition they require, your body begins to break down, symptoms arise, your metabolism slows, and eventually disease develops. The health of your metabolism begins with energy production, and this originates in the deepest part of your cells in the mitochondria. Mitochondria are remnants of small bacteria that symbiotically became part of our human cells. Each cell in the body has about 2,500 mitochondria, which means that more than 1 quadrillion mitochondria exist in our body. This is more than three times the number of human cells and twice the number of our microbiome. Mitochondria are densest in cells that require lots of energy, such as muscle, nerve, and heart cells. Your heart is pumping all day long and requires energy, and even if you are not exercising, your muscles and nerves are still busy at work holding you upright. Nourishing your mitochondria with the proper nutrients is critical for your recovery.

Now, the topic of mitochondrial nutrition belongs more in a masters-level nutrition degree course than in this book; here you'll simply learn the foods to eat to be able to nourish your mitochondrial health back to life. The right foods will increase your energy production, metabolism, lean muscle mass, and fat loss, and they will alleviate pain. Without the right mix of nutrients, your mitochondria will run like my lawnmower—peter out and puff out smoke. Energy will be inefficiently produced, and you will struggle with fatigue, weakness, pain, and weight gain. To produce energy, your mitochondria need oxygen first and foremost—through breathing and exercise (more about this in later chapters). They also need glucose or ketones from fat, along with a mix of vitamins, minerals, nutrients, and antioxidants.

If you eat the right foods, you will nourish your mitochondria and yourself back to health. If you persist for too long in your life deficient in nutrients, mitochondria can even begin to disappear or die off prematurely.

Oxidative Stress

Keeping your mitochondria healthy and maintaining an optimal environment for them to function is essential. When mitochondria do not receive the nutrients they need, especially antioxidants, they can produce something called oxidative stress. Oxidative stress is the production of free radicals or single electrons that can cause cell damage and early cell death. Let's look more deeply at what it means to oxidize. Essentially, a free radical is a molecule or atom that has at least one unpaired electron, making it highly reactive. When an electron is unpaired, it can react with other molecules, causing cell damage. When this occurs at high levels within our body, it's known as oxidative stress. Some free radicals, such as superoxide (created when an electron has been added to an oxygen molecule) are set off deliberately by our immune system to kill foreign invaders in the body. This becomes problematic when the process of inflammation self-perpetuates and begins to cause damage to healthy cells. The free radical nitric oxide also has many useful physiological functions but becomes toxic when overproduced.

Here are a few signs that your body may be experiencing oxidative stress and you may need to nourish your mitochondria more effectively:

- **You have a chronic disease.** Mitochondrial dysfunction can lead to a host of chronic diseases, including diabetes, fibromyalgia, autoimmune diseases, cardiac disease, seizures, migraines, memory and mood problems, and neuropathy, which cause pain and metabolic disturbances.
- **The bulk of your diet consists of high-sugar, starchy foods.** Too much sugar, high-fructose corn syrup, fruit juices, processed foods, and starchy carbohydrates provide little

nutrition, are high in calories, and cause imbalances in your intestinal microbiome.

- **You take a prescription or over-the-counter drug regularly.** Many drugs cause nutrient depletions. The most commonly used in patients who struggle with pain are statin drugs, NSAIDs, glucocorticoids, opioid-analgesics, antacids and medications that lower stomach acid, DMARDS (disease-modifying antirheumaic drugs), antidepressants, metformin, and other diabetes medications.

- **You feel pain and fatigue.** Pain and fatigue are like twisted sisters. Neither is very pleasant and they often appear together. You may have even received a dual diagnosis that incorporates both pain and fatigue, such as fibromyalgia and chronic fatigue syndrome. It's a chicken or egg phenomenon to figure out which one came first. Struggling with one or both is a sign your mitochondria need nourishing. There is also a correlation between chronic headaches and mitochondrial dysfunction.

- **You overexercise.** Overexercise? When I tell patients this, they look at me as if I have ten heads, because they automatically assume more is better. In fact, the wrong exercise or even too much of the correct exercise can lead to oxidative stress. This is often seen with overtraining syndrome in athletes but also in those who are missing vital nutrients from their diet and are overambitious with their fitness goals.

Your Fat-Burning Powerhouse

Energy is vital to your existence, as well as your weight loss and pain management, but the truth is we don't really *create* energy. We *convert* energy by breaking down and using the most basic units stored in our food, which are carbohydrates, proteins, and fats. To be more specific, our body uses glucose found in carbohydrates or free fatty acids from fats to create energy. To create energy, our body has a variety of options—biochemical pathways—available. These pathways existed so

Do You Feel Like the Tin Man?

There is perhaps no better figure to demonstrate what it is like to live in a proinflammatory state with poor mitochondrial health than the Tin Man in *The Wizard of Oz*. The Tin Man rusted from years of rain, environmental exposure, sun, and other factors, so that his joints were stiff, he had trouble moving, and he was in pain. The rust was caused by free radical damage and oxidation. The Tin Man needed just the right amount of oil, as well as some help from Dorothy, who moved his stiff limbs to get his joints working. Now you don't exactly rust like the Tin Man, but your tissues do become inflamed, damaged, and thickened, which leads to stiffness. You've already learned about the oil change to help your pain and stiffness, and in later chapters you will learn about how to get your body moving again after being sedentary and stiff for years like the Tin Man. Focusing on omega-3 fats, monounsaturated fats from olive oil, and medium-chain triglycerides from coconut oil will help eliminate your inflammation and give you energy so you can live an active life.

that as humans we could adapt to different environments and changes to our diet during ancestral times.

You may have heard that your body's preferred source of energy is carbohydrates. Glucose is the simplest form of carbohydrate and most available, due to diets high in carbohydrates, to be used by your mitochondria for energy. The glucose gets stored primarily in two places—your muscles cells and your liver—but the rest of it gets converted into fat and wrapped around your belly. Your body stores glucose in your muscle cells, because muscle cells need immediate access to glucose for fuel. But glucose is also stored in the liver, specifically so that your body has a reserve to feed your brain. Your brain does not have the ability to store energy in any form, so it relies on the liver to send it a steady supply of energy on a consistent basis, all day long and every day.

The truth is that you don't really need all of these carbohydrates for energy, and in fact, years of living with a constant influx of dense or processed carbohydrates in your diet has left you overweight and full of pain. The dense and starchy carbohydrates never get burned up and used for fuel; instead they get packed on your waist and belly and stored as fat. We know now that the fastest way to put on weight and store fat is to consume an overabundance of carbohydrates. Excess carbohydrates are broken down by the body and reassembled as fat and stored as fat tissue.

So, now you know that your body burns glucose first and fast, but what happens after it's all gone? How do you survive? Again, Mother Nature is more evolved than we realize, and our body quickly flips the switch from burning carbohydrates to fat. Glucose is *not* the preferred fuel of muscle cells under normal human resting metabolic conditions, or even under most normal human exercise patterns. Fat is. If given an unlimited supply of glucose and regular refueling (a.k.a. bingeing) of carbohydrates, skeletal muscle will burn through it during exercise the same way a fire burns through a stack of hay. It burns up fast and you run out of it. But skeletal muscle can burn fat with great efficiency and for long periods of time. This is exciting because most of us have plenty of fat reserves on hand to burn and use for energy. The scientific name for this is ketosis. Ketosis is the ability of your mitochondria to switch from using glucose as fuel to using ketone bodies as fuel, and fat is the main source for the production of ketone bodies. Ketones (acetoacetate, acetone, beta-hydroxybutyrate) are available to some degree all day long, but if carbohydrates are unavailable or minimally available, ketone bodies are rapidly created and utilized for energy. The liver immediately shifts to make ketone bodies, so they can be quickly shuttled to the brain for energy. Cardiac muscle actually prefers ketones, and the brain can run just fine (maybe even optimally) on a blend of ketones and minimal glucose.

Our survival as a species has depended on these evolutionary adaptations away from glucose dependency. Entire civilizations have existed for ages on what is practically a zero-carb diet. Think about it rationally—there is very little requirement for any essential dietary carbohydrates in human nutrition. It's possible to live a long and healthy life never consuming much in the way of carbs, provided you obtain adequate and healthy sources of dietary protein and fat, vitamins, and phytonutrients. The same can't be said for going too long without protein or fat. If you cut too far back on either of those macronutrients, you will eventually get sick and experience disease. That is why they are called essential fatty acids and essential amino acids.

Reducing Persistent Pain

Poor mitochondrial health and function have been associated with chronic, persistent pain. Oxidative stress in our cells and mitochondria can lead to muscle fatigue, pain, and tissue damage. Unchecked oxidative stress causes poor energy production, better known and experienced as fatigue. If oxidative stress continues, inflammation will flourish with eventual cell damage. The pain that accompanies inflammation, if left unchecked, will eventually break down connective tissue. This is one reason why sarcopenia, the loss of muscle mass, is seen in patients with persistent pain and why exercise is vital for recovery.

Protecting and enhancing your mitochondrial health and reducing inflammation through better food choices will reduce the triggers of inflammation. As you know, sugar is a common trigger for inflammation and the cause of the increased pain and weight gain you struggle with daily. Remember that sugar is a hidden ingredient in many foods—refer back to the previous chapter for some of its common hiding places. The key anti-inflammatory nutrients that support mitochondrial health are fatty acids EPA and DHA, found in cold water fish and organic, free-range meats, phytonutrients found in vegetables, and antioxidants found in spices. You are still avoiding gluten and dairy in this phase, which often trigger leaky gut, inflammation, pain, and autoimmune-related symptoms. Other vitamins and minerals essential for pain relief include vitamins A, C, D, and B vitamins, calcium, magnesium, manganese, zinc, iron, alpha-lipoic acid, carnitine, resveratrol, and coenzyme Q10, all of which may provide support to your musculoskeletal system function and support. Magnesium and potassium work together to alleviate muscle pain and help with muscle relaxation, tension, and tightness. Maintaining optimal vitamin D levels throughout the year is vital for musculoskeletal pain, especially low back pain and pain caused by migraine headaches.

You Are Now Entering Ketosis

A ketogenic diet is not new and has been used for centuries. I think you now understand how ketosis allowed our ancestors to survive long,

Five Reasons Ketosis Alleviates Pain and Inflammation

There are multiple reasons for the anti-inflammatory effects of a ketogenic diet, and more research is mounting every day. By reading this book and chapter, you are ahead of the curve, gaining the knowledge on how to improve your health. Here are the top five theories summarizing the current rationale:

1. The changes in the brain seen in people who have seizure disorders are very similar in nature to that of chronic pain and thought to involve increased excitability of neurons, both in the central and peripheral nervous system.
2. Reducing glucose metabolism via ketogenic diets has demonstrated clinical improvements regarding metabolic syndrome and insulin resistance.
3. Fasting has been shown to be analgesic; it alleviates and decreases pain. A ketogenic diet is also likely to be as well, as it mimics a fasting state in the body.
4. Ketogenic diets boost a natural chemical in our body called adenosine, which has analgesic or pain-relieving effects. A similar mechanism exists with acupuncture.
5. Very low-carbohydrate diets, such as a ketogenic diet, are better for reducing weight and maintaining weight loss. Weight reduction is one, if not the most important, factor in the elimination of pain in our modern society.

cold winters when there was little food and the food that was available was low in carbohydrates. It is a way of eating that aims to induce nutritional ketosis by restricting carbohydrate intake and balancing daily amounts of fat and protein. A ketogenic diet is *not* a high-protein diet.

Physicians first utilized a ketogenic diet as a way to prevent seizures in children suffering from epilepsy. The benefits of a ketogenic diet gained some significant press in 1994, when Charlie Abrahams, son of Jim Abrahams, began using a ketogenic diet and successfully recovered from daily seizures, after trying all available antiseizure medications and enduring a futile brain surgery. You can use it as an effective tool to lose weight, increase your energy, and, most important, decrease pain.

Ketogenic healing is a therapeutic plan designed specifically for people who have excess body fat, fatigue, and persistent pain.

Ultimately, it is your decision how deep into ketosis you would like to go. For some, beginning with a lower-carbohydrate, ketogenic focus may be enough to drop the unwanted weight and assist in pain relief. However, you may need to change your life and adopt a stricter ketogenic nutrition plan to see true and lasting results. Hang in there with the program; it is well worth the wait, and many find they continue to eat this way on some level as a lifestyle. And those who have strayed find themselves coming back for healing. If consuming animal products, this plan encourages grass-fed meats that might have a higher-quality fat content. That's okay—remember, it's not the fat but the carbohydrates that have been your downfall. Fat will keep you fuller, provide energy, decrease inflammation, and aid in healing!

A ketogenic diet is characterized by high fat, moderate protein, and low carbohydrates. It will deliver an anti-inflammatory, low-glycemic, gluten-free, low-grain, high-quality fats approach to help you fast-track your healing. This shift in macronutrient ratios will cause your body to cleave and burn fat and create ketone bodies, instead of using glucose as its primary source of fuel. Ketones are produced by the liver when fat is burned instead of glucose. The benefit to you is that you will notice that you have sustained energy instead of the roller-coaster highs and lows you once experienced multiple times a day from eating carbohydrates. The best part is that ketones are quickly and efficiently used by all cells of your body, especially your brain and nerve cells, and provide the protective benefit of preventing free radical damage. Ketosis has also been shown to cause mitochondrial neogenesis, which is the production of new mitochondria. This is a good thing. The more mitochondria you have, the more energy you can produce and the healthier you will be.

Five Steps to Ketogenic Healing

To take advantage of the powerful healing properties of ketogenic healing, you need to: (1) consume more fat, (2) cut out carbohydrates, (3) limit your fruit intake, (4) undertake intermittent fasting, and (5) reduce your portions. As you will see, these five strategies have a

How Do I Know Whether I'm in Ketosis?

The first question you need to ask yourself is, "Have I been restricting my carbs?" If you are progressing from my Gut-Healing Protocol, you are halfway there, as you have already been eating a lower carbohydrate diet than usual. However, in this phase, if you think you can cheat with just a little bit of your favorite sweet fruit because it's "healthy," well, I'm here to tell you, you are mistaken. It does take some discipline to achieve ketosis, but believe me, it's worth the effort. The easiest way to test whether you are in ketosis is to purchase urine ketone strips at your local pharmacy. These are inexpensive and readily available, often located in the section with blood glucose monitoring devices. When ketone bodies are present in sufficient amounts, they will appear in your urine, as detected by a ketone strip. Listening to your body's signals is another way to determine whether you are in ketosis, and they include:

- Weight loss
- Increased energy
- Improved mood
- Decreased pain
- Improved focus and concentration
- Feeling full or satiated with meals

Last, when your body enters ketosis, you may sense a sweet smell on your breath, sweat, or urine. Some people refer to this as ketogenic "fruity"-smelling breath, and it is caused by the amount of acetone in your body. If you detect any of these signs, you are more than likely in ketosis.

Isn't Ketosis Bad for You . . . or Is That *Ketoacidosis?*

Although it may sound like they mean the same thing, there is a huge difference between ketosis and ketoacidosis. Nutritional ketosis, also known as physiologic ketosis, is a natural way to shift how your mitochondria produce energy and is a natural biomechanical mechanism available to all. Every person alive enters some form of mild ketosis each time he or she refrains from eating for six to eight hours. *Ketoacidosis* is *not* normal and can be a dangerous and life-threatening metabolic state that occurs in type 1 diabetics, as well as those with the most advanced stages of late-stage type 2 diabetes. It can also affect alcoholics and those with pancreatitis and kidney diseases.

Ketoacidosis occurs when the body is unable to regulate the amount of ketones in the blood and they reach dangerous levels. This can occur in type 1 diabetic patients because they completely lack insulin. Symptoms of ketoacidosis include nausea, vomiting, confusion, and shortness of breath. For anyone who suspects he or she is not in good general health, I recommend consulting a medical professional for guidance with a ketogenic diet.

huge impact on the way your body uses energy, often leading to dramatic weight loss and a noticeable reduction in pain. If you are suffering from persistent pain and appear to be weight-loss resistant, I recommend remaining on this phase for at least three weeks to get your body into an optimal fat-burning state.

First, Increase the Fat

Here is the part most people get really excited about. After *years* of fearing fat, you can now once again enjoy living without the fear that fat in your diet will clog your arteries or make you fat. You now understand that a processed and high-carbohydrate diet—not fat—causes inflammation. Increasing your fat intake is the second-most-important step in achieving a mild state of ketosis (cutting carbohydrates way, way down is number one!), but I put this first because it is the key step most people leave out. They think ketosis is all about cutting the carbs, and you *will* cut your carbohydrates, but you will replace those lost calories with healthy fats. This is why a ketogenic diet is not a starvation diet, and you will feel full and satisfied.

A high-fat, moderate-protein, and minimal-carbohydrate diet will be converted into ketones, which are an excellent source of energy for your mitochondria in muscle, nerve, and brain cells. The majority of your calories will now be derived from fat. I recommend that you aim to obtain a macronutrient ratio of approximately 5 to 10 percent carbohydrates, 20 to 30 percent protein, and 70 percent fats. You do have some flexibility here with the ratios, as the amount of carbohydrates affect everyone differently and so does the fat content, especially medium-chain triglycerides that your body can use to convert to ketone bodies. Use your ketone strips to see how your macronutrient ratios are affecting you personally. Occasionally, you may consume a very small serving of a starchy vegetable or gluten-free grain, but you have to monitor your ketones to know how it is affecting you. This may be needed if you are exercising at a higher intensity. Your body will use fat in place of carbohydrates to create energy derived from ketone bodies, so it is important that you know how to prepare your meals and what you should be eating.

You may feel optimal eating this way because you will have an anti-inflammatory trifecta occurring in your body, consisting of:

1. Healthy omega-3 fats to decrease inflammation
2. Medium-chain fats from coconut products to produce energy via ketones
3. A very low-carbohydrate diet to prevent insulin and blood sugar dysregulation

You are now truly using food as medicine to leverage your healing. I have simplified much of this for you with the recipes flagged for this regimen in Appendix A.

You also have to learn exactly what type of fat to incorporate into your diet. Not all fats are created equal, and this is not an invitation to forget about everything we covered in the previous chapters. Dairy is not allowed back in, because it is way too inflammatory. In addition to healthy omega-3 fatty acids and olive oils discussed in the previous chapters, you will now rely heavily on coconut oil and coconut products, such as full-fat coconut milk, as these will be the easiest way to obtain ketones. Coconut oil contains medium-chain fatty acids, MCTs for short. Your liver will take the medium-chain fats in coconut oil and directly use them as energy and ketone body formation. Medium-chain fats are a powerful source of instant energy to your

Coconut Product Shopping

If possible, you want to purchase organic virgin coconut oil and full-fat, unsweetened coconut milk and coconut butter. These products are more widely available now, as people are aware of the benefit of medium-chain fats in coconut oil and learning how to cook with them. Full-fat coconut milk and coconut cream is a great substitute for dairy, milk, and cheese sauces in many recipes. Light coconut milk does not have enough fat to keep you in ketosis, so make sure to purchase the full-fat kind, which is often sold canned. Be cautious of such products as condensed or other sweetened forms of coconut products. These have added sugars, which will prevent you from reaching ketosis.

body, a function usually served in your diet by simple carbohydrates. Although coconut oil and simple carbohydrates share the ability to deliver quick energy to your body, they differ in one crucial respect: Coconut oil does not produce an insulin spike in your bloodstream. Coconut oil acts on your body like a carbohydrate, without any of the debilitating insulin-related effects associated with long-term high carbohydrate consumption!

Leverage Fat to Get Thin

Fat has long received its bad boy reputation for causing clogged arteries and heart attacks and was practically a four-letter word for most doctors. Here is why that is not true: First, your body needs fat from food to absorb fat soluble vitamins, such as vitamins A, D, E, and K. Absorption of fat-soluble vitamins in the gastrointestinal tract depends on fat for absorption and metabolism. If you have been limiting fat from your diet, you could be causing a deficiency of one of the above vitamins and slowing you metabolism. Next, fat is needed to build the walls of your cells known as cell membranes. The vital exterior of each cell, as well as the sheaths surrounding nerves, are made up of a phospholipid bilayer—basically, rows of fat cells and proteins. Each cell wall in your body is made of mostly fat with some protein. Lipid—that is, fatty—molecules constitute the mass of most cell membranes, nearly all of the remainder being protein. (Now you see why proteins and fats are essential!) Last, fat is needed for muscle movement and decreasing inflammation.

Generally speaking, fats can be broken down into three major categories: saturated, polyunsaturated, and monounsaturated fats. The saturated fats have received the most criticism because people believe that saturated fat in meat causes heart disease, but we need to calm the winds around this controversy. Interestingly, the types of saturated fats that do cause heart disease—stearic and palmitic acid—don't come from meat. Your liver produces these two fatty acids when you eat sugar and carbs. In one interventional trial, researchers revealed that even on a low-carb diet that is higher in saturated fats, blood levels of saturated fats remained lower because of the carb effect. Simply put: In the absence of sugar and refined carbs, fiber and adequate amounts of omega-3 fats in your diet, saturated fat is really not a problem. Again, quality matters: The saturated fat in a fast-food cheeseburger is completely different than what you get in coconut butter or a grass-fed steak. Although you have probably heard the majority of health professionals and the media squawking about how saturated fats are bad for your health and lead to a host of negative health consequences, such as elevated cholesterol, obesity, heart disease, and Alzheimer's disease, in reality the American levels of heart disease, obesity, elevated serum cholesterol, and Alzheimer's have skyrocketed in recent years compared to our ancestors who regularly consumed saturated fats. What has changed? The amount of refined carbohydrates, sugar, and high-fructose corn syrup! In recent years, we have learned more, and new research reveals that saturated fats do *not* cause heart attacks. You can eat them without worry.

Polyunsaturated fats are a bit more devious, but there is a huge difference between processed and natural. Processed polyunsaturated fats (such as margarine spreads and corn, sunflower, safflower, soy, and cottonseed oils) are terrible and inflammatory due to their abundance of omega-6 content, and many also include trans fats. These *do* have a connection with heart disease and should be avoided forever. However, there are naturally occurring polyunsaturated fats in such foods as nuts and seeds, which are great for us and improve cholesterol. It's your job to seek out the healthy fats and eliminate the unhealthy fats.

Last but not least, we have monounsaturated fats. These are also known to be healthy and accepted as having anti-inflammatory effects. Olive oil is a primary example of something that is more proportionately a monounsaturated fat and therefore is healthy for us and lowers our cholesterol.

Then, Cut the Carbs

The only way to achieve a mild ketosis is to dramatically reduce your carbohydrate intake. The low-carbohydrate approach consists of 50 to 80 grams of carbohydrates per day. As caloric needs rise, protein and

Healing Fats	Harmful Fats
Avocado oil	All butter substitutes
Coconut oil	Canola oil
Extra-virgin olive oil	Corn oil
Fat in meat and fish	Grapeseed oil
Fat in nuts and seeds	Margarine
Fish oil	Safflower oil
Flax oil	Soybean oil
Ghee	Sunflower oil
Hemp oil	Vegetable oil
Walnut oil	

fat portions increase. If you are an athlete and burning more calories by participating in intense exercise, you may increase your carbohydrate intake to 100 grams per day. To help guide you, 5 grams of carbohydrate can be found in 1 cup of raw leafy vegetables (about the size of a small fist) or ½ cup of other vegetables.

During the ketogenic healing phase of the Healing Pain Program you will avoid all grains, starchy vegetables, and legumes. I realize you have been told some of these foods provide beneficial nutrients and fiber, but you will be able to achieve the same, if not greater, nutritional benefit from the list of foods provided. There is still variety and nutrient density in the approved vegetables, fruits, protein, and fats allowed. The best types of vegetables for a ketogenic diet are high in nutrients and fiber but very low in carbohydrates. As you can probably guess, these are dark, green, and leafy. Anything that resembles spinach or kale will fall into this category, and you should aim to include these foods in anything you can. But you will also be able to eat such things as broccoli, cauliflower, avocados, and meat and fish.

Limit Fruit

Fruit can be one of the toughest hurdles for people to overcome. Fruit is natural, and it is true that it does have some vitamins, minerals,

Carbohydrates to Avoid

All grains
Fruits
Legumes*
Potatoes

———————

*It is true that beans are a good source of protein and fiber, but they are also packaged along with lots of carbohydrates, and it can be almost impossible to achieve or maintain ketosis if you are eating beans. Beans also contain lectins, which are implicated in nutrient deficiencies, leaky gut, and autoimmunity. If you are very active, you may add one small serving of beans or nongluten grains twice a week while on this protocol. But this is strictly reserved for those who are active, athletic, and performing high intensity exercise, such as in Chapter 9. Typically, this is best achieved with dinner and directly after a workout, as your body will be able to readily use the glucose and you will have the added benefit of fasting for twelve hours as you sleep.

antioxidants, and phytonutrients—all the things you need to fight inflammation and support your mitochondria. However, fruit contains fructose as the main ingredient, which is a sugar. Previously, you could eat apples, pears, or an occasional orange, but here I want you to be a bit more diligent to keep your blood sugar under control. All the berries are allowed, and I encourage you to eat them with some protein or fat. Berries with full-fat coconut milk will slow down the release and absorption of glucose. You can eat a small apple or one quarter of a larger apple as a snack, if you have it with some nut butter, such as almond, hazelnut, or walnut. The fat in the nut butters will help keep ketone production up as well. Limit your fruit to one serving per day.

Nut Butters

Almond	Macadamia
Coconut	Walnut
Hazelnut	

Juice and Dried Fruits

One hundred percent organic juices may be a good source of vitamins, minerals, and phytonutrients, but they do not belong in ketogenic healing. The processing of fruit juice strips it of its natural fiber, leaving behind only the sugar. That's why it tastes so sweet and you can become addicted to it. The dehydration process of dried fruits can be another challenge, as it acts to concentrate the sugars. Let's face it—no one eats one dried apricot!

Implement Intermittent Fasting

If you follow any of the paleo nutrition and fitness communities, you may have read some information online about intermittent fasting. Fasting has been practiced for centuries, but only now are we beginning to understand its effects on inflammation, optimizing energy, and supporting our health. As humans, we now have enough information to reveal that it helps reduce obesity, hypertension, and the pain of rheumatoid arthritis.

One of the aspects that is particularly interesting for those who suffer from persistent pain is the anti-inflammatory effects of intermittent fasting. A number of studies in humans have indicated that intermittent fasting reduces inflammatory markers, such as C-reactive protein and cytokines. The beneficial effects of intermittent fasting (and calorie restriction, which will be discussed later) stem from reduced oxidative damage and increased cellular stress resistance. From an evolutionary perspective, intermittent fasting was probably a regular occurrence for humans. In prehistoric times, there were no supermarkets, restaurants, or convenience stores, and food was not nearly as abundant or easy to obtain as it is today. Nor did we have the kind of predictable eating routine—or should I say overeating routine—we are now accustomed to in our modern world. Our paleo ancestors often went twelve to sixteen hours between meals on a regular basis. At times some may have had to endure full days when they ate very little or ate nothing at all.

According to the journal *Current Pain and Headache Reports*, recent evidence from clinical trials reveals that modified fasting (200–500 calories nutritional intake/day) for periods from seven to twenty-one days is effective in the treatment of rheumatic diseases and chronic pain syndromes. Even better, fasting is frequently accompanied by increased alertness and mood, so fasters feel better mentally. The beneficial claims of fasting are supported by experimental research, which has found fasting to be associated with increased brain availability of serotonin and endogenous opioids, all of which help to alleviate pain. Fasting-induced neuroendocrine activation and mild cellular stress response with increased production of brain derived neurotrophic factor may also contribute to the mood enhancement of fasting. The mood-enhancing and pain-relieving effect of therapeutic fasting is useful as an adjunctive therapeutic approach in chronic pain patients.

The Easiest Way to Fasting: The 12-Hour Fast

You now understand that fasting works some powerful magic when it comes to your health, but understandably, you're not about to live the life of a Tibetan monk or go on a hunger strike for seven-plus days. I don't blame you! Remember, I come from an Italian family, and for me food is fun, family, and enjoyment. But as a good scientist I can't ignore the importance of fasting. The good news is that you can fast every day and not even know you are doing it. As part of the ketogenic healing phase, I want you to fast every day for twelve hours—the majority of which will be done while you are sleeping.

You see, so many of us—due to our lifestyle of long work hours, family, and obligations—don't eat until well after seven, eight, or even nine o'clock at night. For many people, dinner is the largest meal of the day, which means you're going to bed with a belly full of food! Even worse, your digestion never gets a break, and it can be disruptive to your deepest levels of sleep due to blood sugar and insulin changes. And if your body is digesting food throughout the night, it never gets to produce ketones or focus on rest, healing, and rebuilding, which is what sleep is designed to do.

For the next three weeks, I want you to finish eating by seven o'clock in the evening and not eat again until at least seven a.m. the next day. *You can do this.* The key to success is being prepared and knowing what you are going to eat and ensuring that you have it on hand. Most of my clients begin to eat their last meal of the day at six p.m. and are done before seven p.m. Between then and bedtime, you have a few hours to kill, which can be used to relax and get caught up on activities that are not too stressful. That's all you have to do to implement fasting into your life. If you absolutely cannot fit it in, due to work dinners or kid activities, I have seen this work for some people who only fast four days per week. Seven is optimal, but I'll settle for four if absolutely needed. This is better than going on a hunger strike like Gandhi. Our paleo ancestors were sleeping when the sun went down most days, engaging in a natural nightly fast for twelve hours. The sooner we stop eating in the evening, the longer this fast becomes, and the more the body can benefit from it. Like any fasting method, internal energy is freed up that can then be used toward healing the body.

Consume Fewer Calories

One of the wonderful aspects of ketogenic healing is the fact that you will often feel satiated, experiencing less craving and desire to eat. Many people simply feel like eating less, which can be a welcomed bonus, as they have struggled with cravings for years. Long gone are the days where losing weight was solely about cutting and burning more calories. The truth is that the overwhelming majority of people feel hungry when they cut calories, and their willpower eventually disappears, along with the weight they lost. However, since you are in the ketogenic healing phase, you have not one but two distinct advantages to help you decrease your portion sizes a bit: You are continuing with nonstarchy vegetables that are high in fiber, and you are adding more fat to your diet—upward of 70 percent. These two distinct nutritional combinations, along with moderate protein, have worked to provide the advantage of feeling fuller or satiated and for longer periods of time. Without starchy carbohydrates, your blood sugar will remain balanced for longer periods of time, diminishing your cravings.

Research suggests that reducing or restricting calories somewhere by just 20 percent will provide many of the anti-inflammatory and mitochondrial protective qualities you desire to help you heal, lose weight, and decrease pain. The best part is that because of the satiating effects, you will not even notice a 20 percent reduction. Reducing your calories by 20 percent may seem as if you need to understand exactly how many calories you eat at each meal and how many calories are in every food, which can be time-consuming and annoying. Forget that. You'd be surprised that most nutrition professionals don't even know that information and have to rely on fancy computer programs. Simply picture your typical dinner plate and eat about a quarter less. For example, if you usually order the 10-ounce steak, cut it down to 8 ounces, or cut the 6-ounce to 4 ounces. Another way is to take the portion of food you have, cut it in half, and then cut it in half again, leaving out one quarter of the food from your meal. At breakfast, instead of having two jumbo eggs, try having one or two smaller eggs. It's best not to eliminate too many of the vegetables, since they have the highest nutrient density; instead focus on the other items on your plate, such as meats or fish.

Healing Protein Shake

A healing protein shake can still be used in the morning for those of you who like the ease of a morning shake. You can also use a healing protein shake in the evening as a way to reduce calories from your day, if you are feeling satiated, or move toward your evening fast more rapidly. I've included some ketogenic shake recipes in Appendix A.

Seven-Day Ketogenic Meal Plan

This one-week meal plan will help you get started on the ketogenic healing portion of the Healing Pain Program. As you will see, it follows all five steps and incorporates lots of healthy fats, while limiting carbohydrate and fruit intake. See Appendix A for ketogenic recipes.

Meal Timing

In core nutritional healing and gut healing, I wanted you to eat three meals a day, with four to six hours between each meal. Now you can

	Sunday	Monday	Tuesday	Wednesday	Thursday	Friday	Saturday
Breakfast	Poached Eggs with Ghee and Cilantro Ketogenic Coffee or Ketogenic Tea	Chocolate Shake Ketogenic Coffee or Ketogenic Tea	Vanilla Shake Ketogenic Coffee or Ketogenic Tea	Cacao-Mint Shake Ketogenic Coffee or Ketogenic Tea	Berry Shake Ketogenic Coffee or Ketogenic Tea	Chocolate Coconut Shake Ketogenic Coffee or Ketogenic Tea	Eggs with Sausage and Greens Ketogenic Coffee or Ketogenic Tea
Lunch	Grass-Fed Beef Burger (no bun)	Turkey Avocado Wrap	Sweet Italian Sausage with Spicy Broccoli Rabe	Turkey Avocado Wrap	Chicken Avocado Lime Soup	Butter Lettuce Salad with Sardines Creamy Sesame Dressing	Slow Cooker Lamb Stew
Dinner	Macadamia-Crusted Cod Turmeric-Dusted Broccoli and Cauliflower	Shrimp with Coconut Cream Sauce and Zucchini Noodles Brussels Sprouts with Pancetta	Slow Cooker Chicken Curry Roasted Cauliflower with Kalamata Olives and Pine Nuts	Slow Cooker Buffalo Brisket Popeye Spinach Salad with Lemon–Olive Oil Vinaigrette	Green Tea Poached Salmon with Escarole Bitter Greens with Almond Sauce	Steak with Chimichurri Sauce "Creamed" Kale or Spinach	Grass-Fed Beef Burger (no bun) Asparagus Wrapped with Prosciutto

have four to six hours between breakfast and lunch and between lunch and dinner, but you need at least twelve hours between dinner and breakfast. And if you feel full, instead of eating dinner, enjoy a protein shake.

What About Everything in Moderation?

But, Dr. Joe, a little sugar never hurt anyone! It may not affect anyone, but it will someone, *and that someone is you.* You likely have failed most options provided to you by conventional medicine. Your body has every ability to heal by applying these strategies to your life. Some of you may do fine with the strategies you learn in the core nutritional healing and gut-healing chapters. Core nutritional healing is about as moderate as it gets. Notice that there are no Popsicles, doughnuts, or ice-cream sundaes anywhere in the book. Moderation is a one-way ticket to placing your body in metabolic mayhem and most people (including me!) fail when it comes to willpower. Our willpower fails because of the addictive quality of certain foods, especially sugar. Moderation is no more if you want to begin real healing.

Do I Need to Eat This Way *Forever*?

You do not need to be in ketosis all the time and, in fact, you will learn to cycle between ketogenic healing and gut healing. Ketosis is a tool you can add to your nutritional arsenal to heal, alleviate pain, and lose weight. The good news is that often within ten days you will notice dramatic changes, especially in your weight. A 2013 study published in the *Journal of Nutrition* cycled eighty-nine obese subjects between a ketogenic diet and a modified anti-inflammatory diet. The study participants followed a staged diet, with periods of a ketogenic diet for twenty days and an anti-inflammatory diet for four to six months. The subjects enjoyed significant weight loss and body fat reduction, without weight regain. There were also important and stable decreases in total cholesterol, LDL, triglycerides, and glucose levels over the twelve-month study period. A three-week trial of the ketogenic healing phase may be all your body needs. After that, you can follow the guidelines and lessons learned from both the core nutritional healing and gut-healing chapters. You may actually feel so good on this phase of the Healing Pain Program and notice such

Who Should *Not* Be on a Ketogenic Diet?

Those with type 1 diabetes or those suffering from acute adrenal fatigue or exhaustion should not be on a ketogenic diet. Type 1 diabetes is a complex medical condition that requires close monitoring by a physician and medication. Those suffering from acute adrenal fatigue or exhaustion may not see the same weight-loss benefits. And this is not an optimal strategy for women who are pregnant or breastfeeding.

meaningful improvements that you may decide this is the optimal diet for your health and vitality.

Isn't This Just the Atkins Diet Reincarnated?

The Atkins diet gained widespread popularity and shifted Americans' awareness to the benefits of a very low-carbohydrate, ketogenic-style diet. For the first time, the public began to see how carbs were the barrier to their weight-loss efforts and that years of low-fat dieting were a mistake. Many people experienced rapid weight loss for the first time, despite trying many other diet trends. The Atkins diet became a way of life, as people stripped the carbohydrates from their plates. The media fanned the fad-diet flames with such headlines as "Eat Pounds of Bacon and Lose Weight." People used butter, cream, mayonnaise, vegetable oil, or margarine; sustained themselves on the fattiest cuts of pork; and drowned their food in cheese sauce. However, little emphasis was placed on the health-promoting benefits of vegetables and some fruit as the foundation of a healthy diet.

The reason the Atkins diet didn't survive was first that it was void of healthy fats, because people primarily used dairy and the fat in protein as their primary source of fat. Next, there was no emphasis on nutrient-dense foods that would deliver the essential vitamins, minerals, phytonutrients, and antioxidants. Atkins followers may have been consuming plenty of calories, but they were still hungry because their body needed the nutrients.

The Healing Pain Diet Program, unlike the Atkins diet, utilizes healthy omega fats and whole plant sources of mono and polyunsaturated fats, and it takes advantage of medium-chain fats found in coconut oil. People on the Atkins diet and other low-carbohydrate diets cut carbohydrates and replace them with increased protein. Too much protein can raise blood sugar and can make it difficult to achieve ketosis, thus lacking its healing properties. In addition, a high-protein diet is not recommended for many people, and some of these regimens have been linked to certain cancers, such as colon and prostate cancer. Ketogenic healing emphasizes healthy fats and plenty of nutrient-rich vegetables. The carbohydrates you will be eating on this phase of the Healing Pain Diet are healthy leafy greens, dense in phytonutrients.

Cook Your Way out of Pain

Not only is the type of food important for your mitochondrial health but also the way you prepare it. With many conventional cooking practices, fats and carbohydrates interact in a particular way, forming a chemical bond. This marriage of sugar and fat under high heat with poor oils results in something called advanced glycation end products (AGEs). The higher the heat and the browner and crispier the food, the more AGEs are produced and the more oxidative stress occurs in your mitochondria.

AGEs have a variety of negative outcomes, but some of the worst include exacerbating diabetes and atherosclerosis and reducing muscle function, causing stiff joints and even cancer. AGEs are found primarily in meats cooked at very high temperatures, such as frying. Learning a few different and sometimes easy cooking methods can help to decrease them. Sauté instead of fry, cook with moisture over a low flame, poach, stew, and use a slow cooker to reduce AGEs.

Don't want to give up your Saturday night grilled steak? The best part is that adding some herbs, such as oregano, rosemary, and thyme, to grilled meats can prevent some oxidation, because chlorophyll binds to heterocyclic amines. Couple this with a side of leafy greens and you will negate most of the effects of grilling. Most herbs have very low carbohydrate content, so you do not have to worry about their macronutrient effect on maintaining ketosis. And such spices as cinnamon can have blood sugar regulatory effects. Start incorporating more of the following herbs and spices into your diet: basil, rosemary, cilantro, sage, oregano, thyme, marjoram, parsley, garlic, ginger, turmeric, cumin, cinnamon, nutmeg, saffron, sea salt, pepper, and herbes de Provence.

Foods to Avoid for Ketogenic Healing

Dairy

Gluten

GMOs (soy/corn)

Sugar and artificial sweeteners

All grains, legumes, and starchy vegetables

Fruit (except berries eaten with fat, such as coconut milk/cream or
    protein)

Shopping List

Note: Staple items and items used in multiple recipes in Appendix A are listed as is. For items used in only one or two recipes, those recipes are indicated with an asterisk in case you wish to omit that item.

Beverages and Sweeteners

Alcohol-free pure
    vanilla extract
Coffee
Green tea bags
Matcha green tea powder

Raw cacao powder (for shakes
    and desserts)
Unsweetened coconut almond
    milk

Superfoods

Chia seeds (for shakes)
Grass-fed gelatin (for shakes)
Hemp seeds (for shakes)
Raw cacao nibs (for shakes
    and desserts)

Shredded unsweetened
    coconut (for shakes and
    Almond Butter Treats*)

Oils, Fats, Pantry

Arrowroot flour
Canned diced tomatoes
Cider vinegar
Coconut aminos
Coconut flour
Coconut wraps
Distilled white vinegar
Extra-virgin olive oil
Ghee

Kalamata olives
MCT oil (if desired for
    shakes)
Nut butter
Organic coconut oil
Unsweetened canned
    coconut cream
Unsweetened, full-fat canned
    coconut milk

Herbs and Spices

Curry powder
Dried basil
Dried coriander
Dried oregano
Dried rosemary
Dried thyme

Freshly ground black pepper
Ground cinnamon
Ground cumin
Ground turmeric
Red pepper flakes
Sea salt

Nuts and Seeds

Macadamia nuts (for Macadamia-Crusted Cod*)
Pine nuts

Walnuts (for Popeye Spinach Salad* and Coconut Cream Sauce*)

Produce (purchase organic whenever possible)

Arugula
Asparagus (vegetable side)
Bitter greens (dandelion, collard, mustard, chicory; for vegetable side)
Broccoli (vegetable side)
Brussels sprouts (vegetable side)
Butter lettuce (for salad)
Carrots
Cauliflower (vegetable side)
Celery
Cilantro
Cucumber (for shakes and salad)
Escarole (for Poached Salmon*)

Flat-leaf parsley
Fresh mint
Frozen berries (for shakes)
Frozen kale (for shakes)
Garlic
Ginger
Kale (vegetable side)
Lemons
Limes
Oregano
Portobello mushrooms
Red onion (for Spinach Salad*)
Ripe avocados
Roma tomatoes (for Chicken Avocado Lime Soup*)

Romaine lettuce (for burgers
and wraps)
Rosemary
Rutabaga (for Slow Cooker
Lamb Stew*)
Spinach

Summer squash
Turnip (for Slow Cooker
Lamb Stew*)
White onion
Zucchini

Meats and Eggs (purchase organic whenever possible)

Bacon (for Popeye Spinach
Salad*)
Beef or chicken bones
(for broth)
Boneless chicken thighs (for
Slow Cooker Chicken*)
Buffalo brisket (for Slow
Cooker Buffalo Brisket*)
Chicken breast (for Chicken
Avocado Lime Soup*)
Cod fillets (for Macadamia-
Crusted Cod*)
Cooked shrimp (for Shrimp
with Coconut Cream
Sauce*)
Eggs (for breakfast and
Macadamia-Crusted
Cod*)
Ground grass-fed beef (for
burgers)

Lamb stew meat (for Slow
Cooker Lamb Stew*)
Pancetta (for Brussels Sprouts
with Pancetta*)
Prosciutto di Parma
(for Asparagus Wrapped
with Prosciutto*)
Ribeye, skirt, or NY steak
(for Steak with
Chimichurri Sauce*)
Roast turkey breast, sliced
fresh (for Turkey Avocado
Wrap*)
Sausage (for Eggs with
Sausage and Greens* and
Sweet Italian Sausage with
Spicy Broccoli Rabe*)
Wild salmon (for Poached
Salmon*)

Congratulations! You have now successfully completed the Healing Pain
Diet Program. If you have followed it carefully, you should be noticing a dramatic decrease in your pain and significant weight loss,
especially around your midsection. In the next part of the book, we

will focus on the Healing Pain Movement Program, beginning with how to identify what I call Sedentary Syndrome and how to become more attuned to your body—in essence, becoming your own physical therapist. I will help you get your body moving again with a mobility program, which will also have a positive effect on your pain. To learn more about a ketogenic diet, visit www.drjoetatta.com/ketosis.com.

Dr. Joe's Pain Relief Reminders

- If pain persists, a ketogenic diet is one alternative to try for pain relief and weight loss.
- A ketogenic diet shifts your body into a state known as ketosis, where your mitochondria switch from using glucose as fuel to using ketone bodies.
- A ketogenic diet is characterized by high fat, moderate protein, and minimal carbohydrates.
- The five steps to ketogenic healing include: increasing fat, cutting carbs, limiting fruit, implementing intermittent fasting, and consuming fewer calories.

Part III

The Healing Pain Movement Program

8

RETURN TO MOVEMENT

Your body was designed to have smooth, fluid, and pain-free movement. Movement is innate in your creation, and you are entitled to everything a pain-free life offers. To enjoy travel, play, and socializing with others, you need to be able to move with as little pain as possible. This can all be extremely frustrating if you are currently living below your expectations and avoiding activities, recreation, and pleasure due to your struggle with pain. If you think about it, each and every one of us has triumphed from a place of being immobile and needing help. Each of us has at least once in our life already learned what it takes to become stronger, gain mobility, and move without fear of pain or reinjury. And each of you can achieve this again.

You see, you did not come into this world in pain and disabled, but you definitely were not strong and agile, either. Each of us entered the world pretty much the same way. As a soft, gentle baby, you relied 100 percent on the care of someone else, and quite frankly at the time of your birth you could barely lift your own arm! But through a mother's care, you were nourished with proper nutrition and fed your body the essentials it needed to grow. You were also given some help to perform some of the basic daily activities that you now take for granted. Physically, you were mostly baby fat, had very little muscle, and did not even possess enough strength or mobility to feed yourself. Through the developmental phases, you eventually learned to move your arms and legs and roll over onto your belly. Later you began to kneel and crawl. Soon you possessed enough strength that you could sit on your own unsupported. And as your eyes became aware of the surrounding world, your curiosity called for you to explore and move forward with more might—and the idea of walking was born!

No one taught you how to roll, crawl, or walk. It is innate in you as a human being, and the developmental phases were the first physical struggle you overcame. You endured some major physical trial and error to achieve this. Some days you cried because you found yourself flat on your tummy, unable to flip over. Some days you became frustrated because you tried a thousand times to pull yourself to a standing position but just kept falling on your bum (*boop*). And some days you would begin to walk, but after just a few steps you would fall flat on your face—ouch! On average it takes about a year for an infant to complete the developmental stages of motor control and learn how to walk, and this continues until about age three, when running and agility skills are perfected. During the developmental phases, you are practicing balance, coordination, and working on strength and mobility. You are performing movement and exercises that help to shape your nervous and musculoskeletal system. It didn't happen overnight, but by working on it each day you succeeded.

Now, I understand you are not a baby and the adult frame is different, but the same tools that you utilized to learn movement as a baby still exist within you. Unfortunately, an injury or living a sedentary life has actually caused you to move in reverse. Maybe you limp from knee pain, a flight of stairs seems like Mount Everest, or doing simple household chores feels like a boot camp workout, leaving you sore for days. Maybe you rely on others to help you with some of the most basic tasks that most people take for granted. Your joints are stiff each day and quite possibly you rely on a cane for stability. You have lost the ability to run and be agile, and your walking quality as well as distance is decreasing each week and month. You are suffering from our most problematic condition: Sedentary Syndrome. I will highlight the key characteristics of Sedentary Syndrome to help you see whether you fit the model.

In this chapter, I want you to become your own physical therapist—to begin a new paradigm of physical health where you are more in tune with your body. I'd like you to begin to look at your body from a physical perspective—joints, posture, spine—and develop more of an awareness of your body and how it relates to your pain. You may believe that any type of movement is unattainable because of your pain, but it's exactly what you need for a restart. You will access your mobility and ability to perform daily functions with a series of questionnaires that can help you determine your physical status and enable you to track your progress.

What's Missing from Your Annual Physical Exam

One of the great losses in our modern health-care era is the lost art of the physical exam. Time pressures and increasing reliance on technology have contributed to its demise. Currently, the examination your primary care doctor may conduct as your yearly physical consists of basic blood work to check cholesterol, blood pressure, and blood sugar levels. Your physician will listen to your heart and lungs and feel your abdomen to inspect some of your internal organs. He or she will also check your height, weight, and pulse.

If you have had a yearly physical, you are doing more than most, as only about 45 million Americans are likely to have a routine physical this year. However, if you suffer from persistent pain and your problem is physical in nature, someone needs to examine other areas besides your heart, lungs, and blood chemistry. What's missing? The musculoskeletal system. An entire system that directly relates to your pain and weight has been, well, ignored. The optimal structure and function of your musculoskeletal system is necessary for the function of almost every other body system—endocrine, immune, nervous, gastrointestinal, cardiopulmonary, and more. So, why does no one evaluate this yearly, or in more detail? I do believe time is a major factor, as physicians are under serious time and financial constraints due to how our health-care system operates. It's not their fault and something we all need to recognize. The average doctor spends somewhere between eleven and eighteen minutes with a patient, and I can tell you from experience that is nowhere near enough time to complete a thorough musculoskeletal exam.

Over the span of my twenty-year career, I have identified a new syndrome—one that I hope to shed more light on through this book. While evaluating your blood chemistry is important, are we missing the more obvious physical changes that occur when someone struggles with pain and extra weight? Yes. I call this Sedentary Syndrome!

The Risk Factors for Sedentary Syndrome

I have witnessed this new syndrome in thousands of patients and through my work with other clinicians. Its effects can be seen right in front of our eyes without any special tests or blood markers. The key signs of Sedentary Syndrome include central obesity, poor posture, sarcopenia, joint failure, and difficulty with mobility and basic daily life activities. These are the physical manifestations of living for decades sedentary, overweight, and in pain. They are easily observable to each of us, and you don't need to have a doctorate in physical therapy to notice them. You need to have a minimum of three out of five of these key signs for the diagnosis of Sedentary Syndrome. Read through each one and see whether you can identify how many you may have. The more you have, the more likely you are struggling with Sedentary Syndrome and its effects.

Central Obesity

You have learned in previous chapters about the inflammation caused by belly fat. In addition, there are direct biomechanical—or physical—ramifications of carrying too much weight. It is no secret that gravity is ever present, and the more you weigh, the more you will feel the effects of gravity on your joints with the simplest of daily tasks. Weight plays an important role in joint stress, and with more weight, it places stress on joints, especially weight-bearing joints, such as the ankles, knees, hips, and lower back.

Taking a look at your knees is a good place to begin, as many people can relate to having knee pain. When you walk, the force on your knees is the equivalent of one and a half times your body weight. That means that if you weigh 200 pounds, it is like exerting 300 pounds of pressure on your knees with each step. And as you negotiate stairs, the force on your knee can be two to three times your body weight. Walking down stairs is often worse than going up stairs, because you need to decelerate your body weight. Some of these basic movements, such as squatting to pick something up off the floor, can be four to five times your body weight. Every pound of excess weight exerts about four pounds of extra pressure on the knees. So, even people who are only 10 pounds overweight have 40 pounds of extra pressure on their knees; if they are 100 pounds overweight, that is 400 pounds of extra pressure on their knees! If you think about all the steps you take in a day, you can see why it would lead to premature damage in weight-bearing joints.

Knowing your waist circumference is an important measure for you to track your progress. As you lose weight, you will feel less pain and be more active. In Chapter 4, you learned how to measure your waist circumference. Be sure to keep track of this throughout your healing and weight-loss journey.

Waist Circumference

	Men	Women
Low risk	37 inches and below	31.5 inches and below
Intermediate risk	37.1–39.9 inches	31.6–34.9 inches
High risk	40 inches and above	35 inches and above

Poor Posture

Despite what people may think, perfect posture is not straight posture. The ideal spine has developed an S-shaped curve from the base of the skull down to the sacrum to prevent overdue pressure on joints, intervertebral disks, and certain muscles. A sedentary life of inactivity—and especially sitting—can reverse or alter these curves, and this is an invitation for pain. Spine health is much better in the third world, where people have more active occupations and are less sedentary. Many people still sit on the floor instead of in chairs. Sitting on the floor cross-legged and walking as a means of transportation is a better way of life for you physically in comparison to sitting in a chair or in a car.

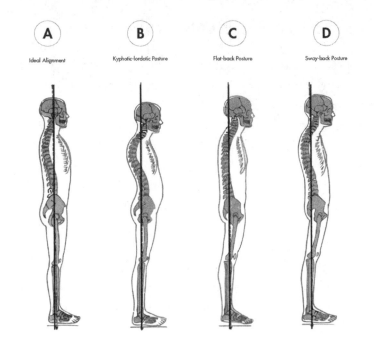

A	B	C	D
Ideal Alignment	Kyphotic-lordotic Posture	Flat-back Posture	Sway-back Posture

Myth: The spine is delicate and easily injured.

Fact: The spine and its surrounding muscles, tendons, and ligaments compose a well-designed structure that's incredibly strong, flexible, and supportive. To help maintain the back and spine, proper conditioning is needed, including strengthening, flexibility, and aerobic conditioning. Although there are some exceptions to the rule (such as an unstable spinal fracture), the back does not need to be overprotected after recovering from a typical episode of back pain.

Oxygen: The Most Important Nutrient

Oxygen is a nutrient? I've never heard that before! Yes, believe it or not, this is the one nutrient most nutrition professionals never talk about. It is an indisputable fact that oxygen is necessary for you to sustain life. Humans can live for days without water, and weeks without food, but without oxygen, cell death begins to occur within three minutes. Your body uses oxygen as its main source of fuel to generate energy in your body. A sedentary lifestyle and the postures you adopt have an effect on how much oxygen is delivered to your lungs.

The Math on Sitting

If you sit and watch television for four hours a day that equals twenty-eight hours each week or two months each year of sitting. In a sixty-five-year life, you will have spent nine years glued to the tube! And once we pass sixty-five, Americans on average watch more than seven hours a day during a time in our life when physical activity is the most crucial! People who watched the most TV in an eight-and-a-half-year study had a 61 percent greater risk of dying than did those who watched less than one hour per day.

A significant portion of our challenges with weight gain and pain can be explained by declining physical activity during the workday. Many people sit for at least eight hours behind a desk and at a computer. This shift translates to an average decline of about 150 calories a day from physical inactivity and is directly affecting our nation's steady weight gain. In total, most people sit for close to twelve hours a day, when taking into consideration their work, commute, and television time.

Sitting will increase your chance of heart disease, cancer, diabetes, and obesity, and it will take years off of your life. A 2010 study in the journal *Exercise and Sport Sciences Reviews* found that even when adults meet physical activity guidelines, sitting for prolonged periods can compromise metabolic health. Simply stated, *too much sitting* is distinct from *too little exercise*. Sitting not only causes you to be in more pain but also affects your metabolism and your efforts to lose weight. Most guidelines by government and health-care officials recommend getting at least 150 minutes a week of moderate-intensity aerobic activity—about 30 minutes a day—or 75 minutes a week of vigorous-intensity aerobic activity, or an equivalent combination of the two. Learning to live a life where you are aware of and consistently try to incorporate small bouts of movement to break up your sedentary day may just be more important than getting 30 minutes daily, as it does not allow your metabolism to slow.

A 2006 report by the American Academy of Physical Medicine and Rehabilitation revealed some striking results based on posture. Using seventy able-bodied participants, the study found that bad posture does indeed affect breathing and lung capacity. They tested slumped seating, normal seating, and standing. They found that slumping produced the worst lung capacity and air flow. No surprise there, given this is what you might expect. Normal sitting was better. Standing posture was the best but not always, as one can have poor posture in a standing position as well. Slumping in a chair is no doubt the worst, but slouching or rounding your shoulders while standing is not much better. Adopting upright postures or, better yet, adapting movement into your life will keep you oxygenated. The mitochondria use oxygen to produce energy, and a lack of oxygen will result in poor muscle metabolism and cause pain.

Your body needs oxygen to be able to:

- Create energy
- Digest food
- Metabolize fat
- Metabolize carbohydrates
- Transport gases across cell membranes
- Manufacture hormones, proteins, and other chemicals
- Regulate pH
- Incite the body to breathe
- Clean and detoxify toxins
- Eradicate virus, amoeba, parasites, fungi, or bacteria
- And much more . . .

Symptoms of poor oxygen include fatigue, an inability to concentrate, brain fog, cravings, muscle tightness and cramping, and, of course, pain. Bringing in fresh air and oxygen is vital to your health, so be sure to adopt a posture that encourages better breathing and air flow.

The Negative Effects of Poor Posture

Sitting causes less demand on the lungs and circulatory system due to the limited mobility. As a result, heart activity and blood flow slow down. And insufficient blood flow, specifically blood that is returning to the heart from the lower legs, causes blood to pool. Pressure on the underside of the thighs from a seat that is too high can further aggravate this situation. The result can be swollen or numb legs and eventually varicose veins. Also, a reduced blood supply to the muscles accelerates fatigue. This is why an employee who sits all day long doing little physical work often feels tired at the end of a work shift.

4 x 4 Breathing for Stress Relief

Due to stress, poor posture, and lack of physical activity, the way you breathe may not be optimal for taking air into your lungs. Healthy breathing is mostly driven by your diaphragm, which causes your belly to pouch out with a deep inhalation and flatten with an exhalation. When you're stressed, your breathing pattern goes haywire. You begin to breathe fast and shallow. You use the muscles in your shoulders, upper chest, and neck instead of your belly. Focusing on deep breathing relaxes the body's stress response, drops the levels of stress hormones, and brings in fresh oxygen.

How to do it: Balancing your breath can do a body good and alleviate stress. To start, slowly inhale for a count of 4, hold for 2 seconds, and then exhale for a count of 4—all through the nose. As you practice and become more advanced, you can aim for a balance of 6 breaths and finally increase to 8 breaths (inhale 8 counts, hold 2, exhale 8 counts). This calms the nervous system, increases focus, and reduces stress.

When it works best: This is one technique that's especially effective when you're in pain or right before bed—the two times when you need relaxation. If you're having trouble falling asleep, this breath technique can help take your mind off racing thoughts and relax you. This also works well in stressful situations or sitting at your desk, to bring in some fresh oxygen!

Limited mobility contributes to injuries in the parts of the body responsible for movement: the muscles, bones, tendons, and ligaments. Another factor is the steady, localized tension on certain regions of the body. The neck and lower back are the regions usually most affected. Why? Prolonged sitting. Sitting reduces body movement, making muscles more likely to atrophy, pull, cramp, or strain when stretched suddenly. It also causes fatigue in the back and neck muscles by slowing the blood supply and puts high tension on the spine, especially in the low back or neck, causing a steady compression on the spinal disks that hinders their nutrition and can contribute to their premature degeneration. Poor posture can lead to a host of health problems, including:

- Spine pain
- Joint pain
- Difficulty walking

- Poor sport performance
- Osteoporosis
- Slowed digestion
- Poor mood or depression

Bad posture also makes you look fatter! When you are slouched over, your internal organs have nowhere to go but down and out—you immediately look larger than you are.

Finally, poor posture worsens stress. Want to relax? Straighten up! A recent study from Harvard University revealed that people who adopted powerful postures (open shoulders and a straight spine) had a 20 percent rise in testosterone levels and a 25 percent decrease in cortisol (the stress hormone). Shallow chest breathing strains the lungs and taxes the heart, as it is forced to speed up to provide enough blood for oxygen transport. The result is a vicious cycle, where stress prompts shallow breathing, which in turn creates more stress.

Sarcopenia

Sarcopenia may just be the biggest health problem you've never heard of. Simply put, sarcopenia, the loss of lean muscle mass and strength, affects an estimated 45 percent of the older US population. From the time you were born to around the time you turned thirty, your muscles grew larger and stronger. But at some point in your thirties, or maybe even your midtwenties if you are inactive, you began to lose muscle mass from sarcopenia. People who are physically inactive can lose as much as 3 to 5 percent of their muscle mass per decade after age thirty. That's a lot of muscle and affects everything from how you look (you know that sagging skin) to how you move. Even if you are active, you will still experience some muscle loss.

Although there is no generally accepted test or specific level of muscle mass for sarcopenia diagnosis, any loss of muscle mass is of consequence, because loss of muscle means loss of strength and mobility. Sarcopenia typically accelerates at around age seventy-five—although it may occur in people aged sixty-five—and is a factor in overall frailty in older adults. It can prevent elderly people from performing the most basic tasks of daily living, and it greatly increases their risk of suffering falls and other serious accidents.

Before we dive into what causes it and how you can prevent it, it's important to understand why sarcopenia can have such a devastating effect on your health. With a loss in muscle mass, the metabolic rate slows down, leading to weight gain and obesity. Reduced muscle mass can also lead to osteoporosis; in fact, one often accompanies or follows the other (though it's clear which one gets the most press). Problems with mobility caused by sarcopenia can result in falls and fractures as well as a loss of physical function and independence. Decreased muscle mass signifies a loss of the metabolic reservoir that would normally help a person recover from illness and surgery, and sarcopenia has been linked to insulin resistance and type 2 diabetes. Older people with sarcopenia are 1.5 to 4.6 times more likely to be disabled than are older people with normal muscle mass. With the many chronic health conditions associated with sarcopenia, it's estimated that a 10 percent reduction in sarcopenia in the US population would lead to $1.1 billion in savings! When you consider its contribution to type 2 diabetes, those savings could be far greater in light of the fact that the annual cost of diabetes is expected to be $192 billion by 2020.

What causes sarcopenia? We may think of decreased muscle mass as a normal part of aging, but a number of preventable factors contribute to sarcopenia, including:

- **Inadequate protein intake:** Amino acids are the building blocks of muscle mass, and we can obtain only certain amino acids (called essential amino acids) from food.
- **Lack of exercise:** Our modern sedentary lifestyle is a huge factor in sarcopenia.
- **Suboptimal hormone levels:** Tissue-building (anabolic) hormones include DHEA, testosterone, and growth hormone. As we age, levels of these hormones decline. If those levels are abnormally low, the body will be unable to maintain lean muscle mass, regardless of how we eat or exercise.

- **Oxidative stress:** An imbalance in oxidant and antioxidant levels can lead to muscle loss.
- **Inflammation:** Infamously known for being at the root of most chronic diseases, inflammation goes hand in hand with oxidative stress and can impact muscle mass directly (through catabolic effects) or indirectly (by affecting growth hormone levels).

Preventing and treating sarcopenia requires an integrated approach that incorporates dietary strategies, hormone regulation, nutritional supplementation, and—most important—exercise. Older adults should strive to ensure an adequate intake of high-quality protein and reduced intake of grains. Because hormonal factors can significantly affect muscle mass, all adults over the age of forty should undergo annual blood testing to track their hormone levels. Regular exercise, particularly weight training, is essential for preserving and increasing muscle mass (more on this in the next chapter). In addition to building muscle, resistance or strength training promotes mobility, enhances fitness, and improves bone health.

Nutrients to Prevent Sarcopenia

- Protein
- Creatine
- Vitamin D
- Omega-3 fatty acids
- Carnitine
- Glutamine
- Coenzyme Q10 (CoQ10)

Joint Failure

Joint failure is another common indication that you may have Sedentary Syndrome. Most people develop joint failure from arthritis, or arthritis-related conditions, such as osteoarthritis, rheumatoid arthritis, gout, or lupus. In fact, joint failure and arthritis are intimately connected: The word *arthritis* encompasses more than one hundred rheumatic diseases and conditions that affect your joints and their surrounding tissues, causing inflammation that leads to pain, aching, swelling, and stiffness in the joint area. Some conditions, such as osteoarthritis, are due to cartilage loss in your joints. Other conditions, such as rheumatoid arthritis, stem from issues in your immune system, causing your body to attack itself. Arthritis is actually more prevalent in people who have heart disease, diabetes, metabolic syndrome, and high blood pressure. Perhaps most interesting to our link between pain and weight gain, 31 percent of people who are obese also develop arthritis. Not surprising, obese adults with arthritis are more physically inactive.

A whopping 52.5 million American adults have been diagnosed with some form of arthritis. While arthritis steadily rises as we age, nearly two thirds of those who have arthritis are actually younger than age sixty-five, and it affects more women than men. Arthritis is on the rise—not surprising when you look at the obesity rates—and government statistics predict that, by 2030, 67 million American adults will have it. Osteoarthritis, the most common type of arthritis, affects millions of people and is caused by aging joints, injury, and obesity, most commonly found in the knees, hips, spine, or fingers.

Nocebo Alert! Negative Thoughts Can Make Arthritis Worse

The nocebo effect is an adverse reaction experienced by a patient. Conversely, a placebo is an inert substance or form of therapy that creates a beneficial response in a patient.

X-rays are useful tests to confirm a diagnosis of osteoarthritis, although they often aren't needed and can cause harm. The brain's processing of such words as *arthritis*, *degeneration*, or *degenerative changes* can be enough to cause or increase pain. This reaction is a nocebo effect. The truth is that many people with awful-looking X-rays of their knees, hips, and spine have absolutely no pain. X-rays may show changes, such as osteophytes, narrowing of the space between bones, and calcium deposits within your joints. X-rays aren't a good indicator of how much pain or disability you're likely to have—some people have a lot of pain from minor joint damage, but others have little pain from severe damage. It is normal for our joints to show signs of aging. As long as it is happening slowly with the hands of time, it shouldn't prevent you from moving and being active.

Arthritis-Related Surgeries

In 2011, doctors performed the following surgeries:

- 757,000 knee replacements
- 512,000 hip replacements
- 76,000 shoulder replacements
- 25,000 other joint procedures

Most of these stemmed from arthritis, which often causes falls and injuries.

What can you do to avoid the joint failure connected to arthritis? Well, some risk factors, such as age and gender, are unchangeable. However, other risk factors, such as excess weight, are within your control to change. If you already have arthritis, engaging in physical activity, watching your weight, and protecting your joints—for example, avoiding repeated knee bending—can help improve your situation. Physical activity is extremely important and people with arthritis are encouraged to perform some type of moderate exercise for thirty minutes at least five times a week. According to research, those with arthritis are often less physically active than those without it. But while many people fear that physical activity will increase their pain or worsen their symptoms, the reverse is true, and even a modest weight loss can dramatically diminish pain and disability. Ideal forms of exercise include walking, bicycling, and gentle strength training. If your pain is the result of some form of arthritis, make sure you are getting enough exercise and get serious about weight loss if you really want to alleviate your symptoms.

The Stiff Facts

- In the United States, 22.7 million people report limitations due to their arthritis.
- 8 million people have difficulty climbing stairs.
- 11 million people can walk only short distances.
- People with arthritis can reduce and sometimes even eliminate symptoms by following the exercise strategies in this book and following the Healing Pain Diet.

Difficulty with Mobility and Basic Daily Life Activities

If you are experiencing restricted mobility, it may be temporary or more permanent, but the more you learn about your physiology through nutrition and muscular activity, the better you will be at adapting and recovering faster. Mobility is also related to changes in your body as you age. Loss in muscle strength and mass, less mobile and stiffer joints, as well as gait changes affect your balance and may significantly compromise your mobility. Mobility is crucial to the maintenance of independent living; if your mobility is restricted, it may affect your activities of daily living. Often we take for granted our physical independence, and it's not until we lose it that we realize the value it contributes to our life. If you have had mobility issues for a while, you may even forget the things you used to be able to do pain-free and with ease. That's normal, but I want you to take a moment to think about when you were the best in your life and the types of activities you used to enjoy.

Now, obviously, if you are ninety years old, no one is going to be able to wave a magic wand and return you to your ballet days when you were sixteen. But you are likely somewhere between forty and sixty years of age and have been struggling with a condition for a few years to a few decades. It's my job to give you the basic education, inspiration, and treatment you need to become fully functional in your life and not fear the physical.

Some of the more common daily problems you may be experiencing involve:

- **Basic activities of daily living,** such as bathing, dressing, toileting, transfers, and feeding
- **Normal daily activities,** such as walking, stairs, travel, shopping, food preparation, housework, exercise, and laundry
- **Advanced daily activities,** such as recreation, sports, play, sports-specific activities, and physical labor

I have included four tests you can use to assess your own physical status, based on a particular body part that may be giving you

Infrared Saunas for Mobility and Pain Relief

Infrared saunas are an effective tool that can help you naturally reduce pain and inflammation. Infrared light (experienced as heat) has the ability to penetrate human tissue to produce a host of health benefits. Infrared heat reduces muscle spasms and helps the body heal itself naturally.

A 2013 study conducted at Auburn University at Montgomery compared stretching in a Sunlighten 3-in-1 sauna compared to a typical environment. Participants completed a series of hamstring stretches in random order with forty-eight hours separating the sessions. Results showed flexibility increased up to three times in the sauna than without! Benefits to the increased range of motion include joint mobility, less friction in the joints, enabling of joint function to diminish stiffness, and joint relaxation.

Sunlighten 3-in-1 saunas have a program specifically for pain relief that uses a blend of near, mid, and far infrared waves to penetrate the muscles and tissues, detoxification, increasing circulation, and speeding oxygen flow. Saunas can be an integral part of a rehabilitation program for chronic fatigue syndrome, fibromyalgia, arthritis, and other chronic pain conditions.

difficulty. Often we ignore pain in hopes that it will go away or we are not sure when to seek help. Waiting too long to intervene on a joint or joints that are painful can hinder your recovery and make pain more difficult to treat. Some of you may have more than one problem area, or if you have a more global condition, such as Parkinson's disease or multiple sclerosis, you may need the Pain and Movement Assessment from Chapter 4 (see page 60). In terms of your overall pain, I want you to rate your pain in the last 24 hours on a scale of 0 to 10, where 10 is pain as bad as it can be. Rate your pain this way every day, so that you can keep track of how you are feeling and improving as you advance through the Healing Pain Program.

New Year, New You?

For so many people, the New Year is a time to reevaluate, and that often includes health and weight loss. I bet you may have made New Year's resolutions to join the gym and finally lose the weight that is

Functional Upper Extremity Exam

Circle "Yes" or "No" next to the following questions, which measure functional activity.

1. Do you have shoulder, arm, or hand pain? Yes No
2. Do you have problems washing your back? Yes No
3. Do you have problems with household chores? Yes No
4. Do you have difficulty typing or writing? Yes No
5. Do you have difficulty opening jars? Yes No
6. Do you have difficulty with activities at work? Yes No
7. Do you have numbness or tingling in an arm or hand? Yes No
8. Do you have difficulty carrying bags, such as groceries? Yes No
9. Does pain disturb your sleep? Yes No
10. Does pain interfere with recreation, sports, or exercise? Yes No

This test will help you assess whether pain in your shoulder, arm, or hand is interfering with your daily life. If you answered yes to three or more questions, it is an indicator you should seek care, such as physical therapy, for your pain or injury.

Functional Lower Extremity Exam

Circle "Yes" or "No" next to the following questions, which measure functional activity.

1. Do you have pain anywhere along your leg (hip, knee, foot)? Yes No
2. Do you have pain or limp while walking? Yes No
3. Do you have pain or limp up/down stairs? Yes No
4. Do you have pain or difficulty squatting to the floor? Yes No
5. Do you have pain or difficulty running? Yes No
6. Do you have pain or difficulty hopping? Yes No
7. Do you have numbness or tingling along your leg? Yes No
8. Do you have pain or difficulty standing for prolonged periods? Yes No
9. Does pain disturb your sleep? Yes No
10. Does pain interfere with recreation, sports, or exercise? Yes No

This test will help you assess whether pain in your leg (hip, knee, foot) is interfering with your daily life. If you answered yes to three or more questions, it is an indicator you should seek care, such as physical therapy, for your pain or injury.

Functional Lower Back Exam

Circle "Yes" or "No" next to the following questions, which measure functional activity.

1. Do you have pain along your lower back, buttock, or down your leg?	Yes	No
2. Do you have pain with or avoid walking?	Yes	No
3. Do you have pain with or avoid stairs?	Yes	No
4. Do you have pain with/avoid daily activities (lifting, care, housework)?	Yes	No
5. Do you have pain with or avoid prolonged sitting?	Yes	No
6. Do you have pain with or avoid prolonged standing?	Yes	No
7. Do you have numbness or tingling down your leg, shin, or foot?	Yes	No
8. Do you have pain with or avoid travel?	Yes	No
9. Does pain disturb your sleep?	Yes	No
10. Does pain interfere with recreation, sports, or exercise?	Yes	No

This test will help you assess whether pain in your lower back or leg is interfering with your daily life. If you answered yes to three or more, it is a sign you need rehabilitative care for your pain or injury.

holding you back from living the life you so desperately want. But here's the thing—if you are significantly overweight and have joint pain, the gym may actually not be the best place for you. Too many people begin exercising or attending fitness classes that are at a much higher intensity than their body can reasonably handle in this state. The gym is not meant for people who have been out of shape for years, and my guess is that the thought of going to a gym probably makes you a bit uncomfortable—for a reason.

So, where should you start? The best place to begin your transformation is in a safe, reassuring, appropriate environment, such as a physical therapy clinic, where you will learn how to exercise and move properly. A physical therapist will be able to slowly work your muscles and joints so that you gradually build your strength, balance, and fitness level, as well as your confidence. You can and *should* still exercise,

Functional Neck Exam

Circle "Yes" or "No" next to the following questions, which measure functional activity.

1. Do you have pain along your neck, shoulder, arm, forearm, or hand?   Yes   No
2. Do you have pain with personal care (washing, dressing, grooming)?   Yes   No
3. Do you have headaches or migraines?   Yes   No
4. Do you have pain with or avoid reading?   Yes   No
5. Do you have pain with or avoid driving?   Yes   No
6. Do you have pain with or avoid using the computer?   Yes   No
7. Do you have numbness or tingling down your arm, forearm, or hand?   Yes   No
8. Do you have pain that interferes with your work?   Yes   No
9. Does pain disturb your sleep?   Yes   No
10. Does pain interfere with recreation, sports, or exercise?   Yes   No

This test will help you assess whether pain in your neck or arm is interfering with your daily life. If you answered yes to three or more, it is a sign you need rehabilitative care for your pain or injury.

even if you are struggling with joint pain, arthritis, problems walking, or a disability. Exercise is vital to your recovery, and the right movements can actually help alleviate your chronic pain. A physical therapy mobility program is a safe place to start, where you won't injure yourself or exacerbate your pain.

How Do I Find a Physical Therapist?

Your ability to visit a physical therapist and how much of your session is covered depends upon your personal health insurance program. That said, in every state there is some form of direct access, which means that you can see a doctor of physical therapy without approval from your physician first. More and more physical therapists are beginning to work with people who fall into the category of not being fully able-bodied but not necessarily having suffered a specific injury. You can find a physical therapist by visiting www.moveforwardpt.com.

WALK Before You Run

Too many people make the mistake of starting an exercise program at full intensity and then burning out quickly because they hurt themselves, are in too much pain, or can't psychologically handle the idea of such a hard, long workout. Nearly two thirds of adults in the United States who make New Year's resolutions have set fitness goals as part of their resolution. Of those, 73 percent gave up before meeting their goal. Remember, you have to walk before you run—sometimes literally! If you begin slowly and steadily increase the intensity of your program, you are more likely to succeed and stick with it.

Progressive Muscle Relaxation

Getting your body to relax is one of the most crucial aspects in the healing process and is a great place to start when you are first beginning a movement program. Muscles can become tense, tight, and stiff from the stress of daily life. When this occurs, pain is not too far behind. Many people go through life every single day and do nothing toward relaxing their body. Progressive muscle relaxation relaxes your muscles through a two-step process. First, you systematically tense particular muscle groups in your body, such as your thigh or neck muscles. Second, you release the tension and notice how your muscles feel when you relax them. This exercise will help you lower your overall tension and stress levels. It can also help reduce physical problems, such as neck pain, back pain, and headaches, as well as improve your sleep.

Step 1: Tense specific muscles. The first step is learning to apply muscle tension to a specific part of the body. Focus on the target muscle group—for example, your left hand. Next, take a slow, deep breath and squeeze the muscles as hard as you can for about 5 seconds. It is important to really feel the tension in the muscles, and it may even cause a bit of discomfort or shaking. In this instance, you would be making a tight fist with your left hand.

Step 2: Relax the tense muscles. This step involves quickly relaxing the tensed muscles. After about 5 seconds, release all the tightness from the tensed muscles. Exhale as you do this step. You should feel the muscles become loose and limp, as the tension flows out. Take time to notice the difference between the tension and relaxation. This is the most important part of the whole exercise. Learning what a tense muscle feels like and a relaxed muscle feels like will serve you in many areas of life.

During this exercise, you will be working with all the major muscle groups in your body. Begin with your feet and systematically move up to your shoulders and neck. Try to relax all of the following muscles in your body:

- Foot (curl your toes downward)
- Lower leg and foot (tighten your calf muscle by pulling toes toward you)
- Entire leg (squeeze your thigh muscles while doing above)
- Repeat on other side of your body
- Hand (clench your fist)
- Entire right arm (tighten your biceps by drawing your forearm up toward your shoulder and "make a muscle," while clenching your fist)
- Repeat on other side of your body
- Buttocks (tighten by pulling your buttocks together)
- Stomach (tighten your stomach and press your back flat)
- Chest (tighten by taking a deep breath)
- Neck and shoulders (raise your shoulders to touch your ears)
- Mouth (open your mouth wide enough to stretch the hinges of your jaw)
- Eyes (clench your eyelids tightly shut)
- Forehead (raise your eyebrows as far as you can)

Once you have become familiar with the two tension and relaxation techniques and have been practicing them for a couple of weeks, you can begin to practice a very short version of progressive muscle relaxation. This can be done at work or home in brief sessions to help you alleviate tension, tightness, and pain.

Ruth: Healing Is Possible

Early one morning, Ruth called her daughter to report that she could not get out of bed and that her legs were "leaking fluid." She screamed into the phone that her knee pain was excruciating! When I met Ruth, she could barely walk and needed assistance plus the help of a walker to transfer to common places, such as the toilet and bathtub, due to safety issues. Her diagnosis was lymphedema of the legs caused by obesity. Ruth had just spent a week in the hospital for the treatment of cellulitis, a common bacterial infection of the skin that had spread to her right knee. Ruth was borderline diabetic with significant blood sugar issues and circulation problems, which caused edema in her lower leg, ankles, and feet. This chronic swelling can cause skin to crack, leaving the skin vulnerable to bacterial infections. She was treated with antibiotics, placed on a low-carbohydrate diet, and given physical therapy. Ruth chose to be discharged to her home instead of an inpatient rehab facility. She lived alone and had a 24-hour home attendant. Upon her discharge from the hospital, it was determined that Ruth weighed 227 pounds, placing her close to the obese category, and she had had enough of living a life confined to her home. She was motivated and ready to make changes.

Ruth admitted that she was always a bigger woman, but after losing her husband to cancer, she let herself go and ate for comfort and to erase the emotional pain. I saw Ruth for physical therapy three times per week for four weeks and then decreased to two times per week for five weeks. Ruth knew she needed to lose weight, as her pain and disability now had confined her to home. At each visit, I would instruct her on exercises to strengthen her legs, work on balance, and improve her ability to walk. I would leave her with a series of exercises she had to do daily, and I instructed her home health aide on how and when to do them with her to give her support and accountability. I continually encouraged Ruth to stick with her exercises and dietary recommendations and even enlisted the help of her two daughters, who did not live with her but who were in constant contact by phone. She knew if she could follow through that in a few months her circulation would improve.

Ruth was compliant with her diet, her circulation improved, and she left behind her daily habit of sitting in her recliner all day to watch television. As her strength returned and her knee pain subsided, her walking improved and she was able to perform the simpler tasks, such as tying her shoes and bending down to put on her pants. She could even squat down to the floor to do simple things, such as cleaning or picking up something she dropped. Her strength improved dramatically, the swelling decreased, and she transitioned rapidly from a walker to a cane and then eventually to walking independently. With her renewed independence, she rejoined her church choir and attended weekly rehearsals and monthly performances, which required her to stand for two hours and have sufficient energy. The best part was that she was able to return to an activity she loved and be surrounded by a community of like-minded people who shared a similar passion.

So much of healing is about your commitment and determination. Ruth's resolve to lose weight and regain her mobility definitely contributed to her success, and I know it can help yours, too. Whatever the cause of your pain, you can—and will—feel better if you commit to doing whatever it takes to help your body heal.

10-Step Personalized Physical Exam

If no one is looking at your movement, I want to provide you with a way you can quickly screen it yourself to obtain a baseline. Any good physical therapy program will include core stability exercises, an emphasis on correct posture, assessing your joint range of motion and flexibility, and increasing balance and coordination. I want you to think about these core concepts as you assess your own range of motion.

The following are ten quick and easy ways to help you determine whether you have problems with some of the most basic foundational and functional movements that you need to be able to perform for most daily activities and even some recreation and sports. This is a general mobility program that you can begin doing yourself at home to slowly get your body moving again.

These mobility exercises engage different parts of your body, including your cervical spine, neck, lower back, shoulders and hips, and feet and hands. They will give you a strong sense of where you feel weak and may need to work harder. Relearning healthy movement patterns that you lost decades ago is the foundation of physical health.

1. Squat

Stand with your feet just wider than hip distance apart. Extend your arms out straight so they are parallel with the ground. Slowly bend your knees until your body is in a squat position. Keep sending your hips backward as your knees begin to bend. While your butt starts to stick out, make sure your chest and shoulders stay upright, and your back remains straight. Keep your head facing forward with eyes straight ahead for a neutral spine. Optimal squat depth

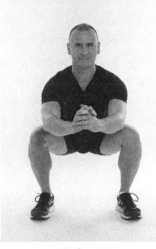

1. Squat

would be your hips' sinking below your knees (if you have the flexibility to do so comfortably). Return to a standing position.

2. Lunge

Start with your feet together in a standing position. Keep your upper body straight, with your shoulders back and relaxed, and your chin up (pick a point to stare at in front of you so you don't keep looking down). Step forward with one leg, lowering your hips until both knees are bent at about a 90-degree angle. Make sure your front knee

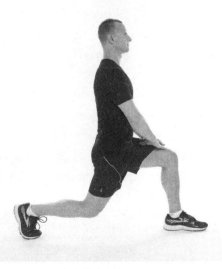

2. Lunge

is directly above your ankle, not pushed out too far, and make sure your other knee doesn't touch the floor. Keep the weight in your heels as you push back up to the starting position.

3. Single Leg Balance

Stand up straight and lift one leg modestly off the ground, balancing on the other leg. Your foot can be either in front or behind you. You may need to have a chair nearby to hold on to at first. Try to balance for at least 10 seconds without putting your foot down for a balance check. Repeat on the opposite side.

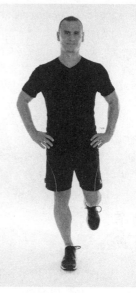

4. Spinal Flexibility

In this exercise you will move from the child's pose position and into a press-up

3. Single Leg Balance

position, testing the full range of spinal flexibility. Kneel down on a mat and bend your body down to the ground with your arms out straight in front of you, stretching out your spine. Then straighten out your legs behind you, place your arms shoulder distance apart in front of you, and curve upward.

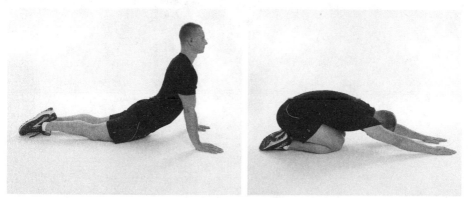

4. Spinal Flexibility

Yoga and Pilates

As you complete a physical therapy program, you may want to transition to an environment where you can continue to focus on your movement and mobility. I often recommend incorporating some type of movement exercise, such as yoga or Pilates, into your routine, because it is an excellent way to shift from a supervised physical therapy program to being more independent. Both yoga and Pilates have been proven beneficial for those with musculoskeletal pain syndromes. You can either take a private lesson or join a group class. Aim to take a class twice per week. This may be a good way for you to advance from physical therapy to some of the concepts we will talk about in the next chapter. Yoga and Pilates both focus on retraining healthy movement and mobility. The missing link you will find with both yoga and Pilates is that unless you perform it at a superadvanced level, it is not efficient at strengthening or rebuilding muscle. More on that in Chapter 9!

5. Plank

Lie down on your stomach on a mat with your legs straight out behind you and push yourself up on your heels and straighten your arms, so that you are supporting your body in a plank position. See how long you can hold this position. Try to hold for 20 seconds.

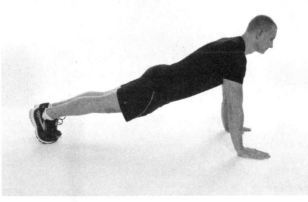

5. Plank

6. Trunk Stability

From the hands and knees position, straighten your left leg behind you while lifting your right arm reaching forward. Support yourself with one arm straight down and the other stretched out in front of you. Your body should essentially be parallel to the ground. Hold for a maximum of 10 seconds and then repeat on other side.

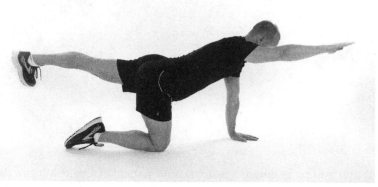

6. Trunk Stability

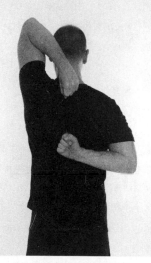

7. Shoulder Flexibility

Stand up straight and lift your left arm above your head, then bend your elbow, and position your hand behind your neck. Bend your right arm and bring it behind your back. Now try this with the opposite arm.

7. Shoulder Flexibility

8. Heel Sit

This exercise tests the mobility of your knees, feet, and ankles. Kneel down on a mat and then lower your body back, so that you are resting your butt on your feet. You should be able to comfortably sit in this position for one minute without pain.

If you have knee or ankle problems, you may need to ease into this exercise.

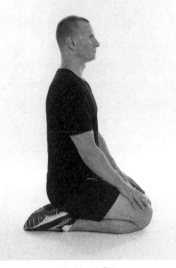

8. Heel Sit

9. Sit-Rise Test

The sit-rise test is an easy test first published in the *European Journal of Cardiovascular Prevention*. Researchers found that the rates of mortality between test subjects differed by quite a great deal, even when controlled for gender, age, and body mass index. The test provides an efficient prediction of mortality risk in elders. In one study of subjects between the ages of fifty-one and eighty, those who had the lowest score range were five to six times more likely to die within the study period (about six years) than were those in the group with the highest scores. This shows you why good mobility combined with strength is so important.

Stand up straight in the middle of the floor with bare feet. It helps if you are wearing comfortable clothes with some give. Make sure you give yourself plenty of space. Cross your legs and gradually lower yourself into a sitting position on the floor, without using any aids, but purely through your own balance. Your feet should be crossed in front of you when the movement is complete. Then try to stand back up, without relying on your hands, knees, forearms, or legs.

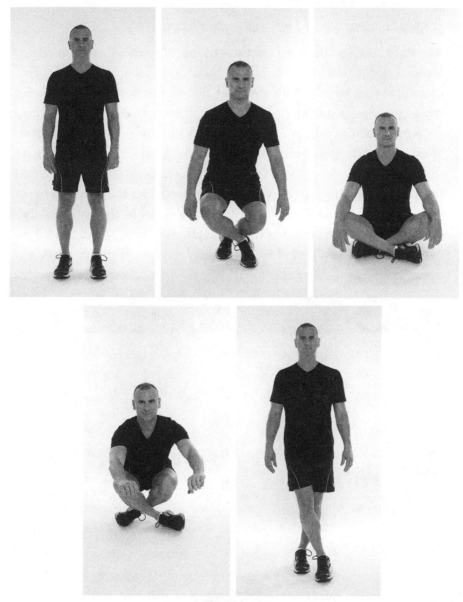

9. Sit-Rise Test

You should be able to get up and down from the floor without the support of your hands.

WARNING: Do not attempt if you are worried the exercise may cause you injury or you are at risk for falls.

30-Second Chair Stand Test (only if you can't do #9!)

Already know you can't get on the ground? Try the 30-second chair stand test. Sit in a chair with your hands on the opposite shoulder crossed at your wrists. With your feet flat on the floor and your back straight, rise to a standing position and sit back down, repeating this movement as many times as you can for 30 seconds. Do not use your arms to stand. If you are more than halfway to a standing position when the 30 seconds are up, count it as a stand. The 30-second chair stand test is another way to measure your leg strength and endurance to predict your likelihood of falls. Healthy people between the ages of sixty and sixty-four are expected to stand and sit more than twelve times for women and fourteen times for men in sixty seconds. If you are younger than sixty, you should be able to attempt the sit-rise test.

Age	Men	Women
60–64	<14	<12
65–69	<12	<11
70–74	<12	<10
75–79	<11	<10
80–84	<10	<9
85–89	<8	<8
90–94	<7	<4

Practice These Exercises

Take the time to try to work through the ten-step physical exam alone or with a supportive partner. It is likely you will have some difficulty getting in and out of a few of the positions. That is normal and can often be solved with a few mobility exercises or yoga a few times a week. Look at this mobility program as easing yourself back into careful movement and exercise and work at it regularly. A good starting point would be to perform the exercises twice a week. Being more active in general will help as well. If, however, you find extreme difficulty, pain, or notice how one test negatively affects your physical function, this may indicate you should see a physical therapist for a full evaluation and treatment. If many of the positions are impossible, it may prevent you from beginning and achieving even the most basic of exercise programs. Once you are able to perform all of the core mobility exercises comfortably, you are ready to move on to a slightly more intense strength-training program.

Hopefully, you now truly believe that you can return to a more mobile and independent state, performing many of the activities you were once able to do without thinking. Understanding the risk factors for Sedentary Syndrome and doing what you can to counteract them will have a huge impact on your movement and pain management. The first step to healing your body is getting it moving again, and you should be able to handle most daily activities, such as shopping and housework. The tests will give you a clear idea of your range of motion and are a great tool for measuring your progress. Once your overall mobility has improved, you're ready to strengthen your body with a more formal exercise program and burn some serious fat with high intensity interval training.

Dr. Joe's Pain Relief Reminders

- The risk factors for Sedentary Syndrome include obesity, poor posture, sarcopenia (muscle loss), joint failure, and challenges with mobility and activities of daily living.
- The gym may not be the best place to begin your movement program; consider physical therapy, which provides a safe and more appropriate environment.
- WALK before you run. Exercise is an essential part of pain relief. Begin where you can and progress steadily but in a pain-free way. An exercise progression is vital.
- Addressing an old injury or a joint that causes you problems is necessary before embarking on a fitness program.

9

STRENGTHEN AND REVITALIZE

I **know what you're** thinking: *You're going to tell me I need to strengthen my body, when the reality is most days I can barely move without feeling pain and fatigue? And do you have any idea how difficult it can be to lift weights with all this extra tissue around my midsection and hips?* I understand, but you are not alone. All of my patients have had those very same challenges, and yet they all began to slowly strengthen their muscles and were surprised by how much better they felt. Exercise actually helps heal your body and reduce your pain. And isn't that what you most want? To have less pain and feel better? You, too, can overcome this belief, which keeps you trapped in an overweight and pain-ridden body, and continue the healing process.

In this chapter, we'll look at exactly why strength training is vital to your healing and how it can help you lose weight much more quickly and optimally than endurance exercises, such as running and biking. And what you may not realize is that strength training is actually cardiovascular as well, so while you're building those muscles, you're also raising your heart rate. Strength or resistance training has so many benefits beyond weight loss—it can increase bone density, reverse sarcopenia (muscle loss), and improve your overall movement and balance, making even everyday activities easier for you. Exercise also has positive effects on your hormones, which help repair muscle tissue, strengthen joints, and grow nerves. Once you realize just how important strength training is, I know you'll want to try it, so this chapter also includes simple exercise programs you can follow, ranging from beginner to intermediate to advanced. So, keep reading and don't give up!

Francine: Healing Is Possible

Francine came to me after being immobilized in a back brace for six weeks. One day while she was bending over to lift the groceries out of the trunk of her car, she heard (and felt!) a cracking sensation in her back and experienced immediate pain that left her doubled over in the parking lot. Francine was sixty years young but had struggled with rheumatoid arthritis and was already on the latest and greatest drug to slow her bone loss. Her lifestyle was completely sedentary; she was fearful of doing any exercise that might hurt her. People often avoid "exercise" but do not realize that most of the daily activities they do, such as cleaning the house and lifting groceries out of a car like Francine, can be just as physical—if not more so—than a properly prescribed exercise program. Francine sustained a compression fracture at her T12 vertebra, just from performing simple daily activities.

Francine's muscles were weak, atrophied, and provided her spine with no strength or stability. She was sedentary and overweight and the straw that broke the camel's back, literally in her case, was the development of osteoporosis in her spine. Furthermore, she had been given a number of glucocorticoid treatments over the course of her life to treat rheumatoid flares, and one of the side effects of these drugs includes thinning bone. Francine *needed* to get stronger because her function was becoming severely compromised. She reported problems with basic daily activities, such as stairs, lifting, and walking, well before her fracture.

When I told Francine that I was going to start her on a resistance-style weight-training program to rebuild the muscle she had lost in her arms, legs, and torso, she expressed concern that she would hurt herself. One of the primary fears or concerns of many patients is that they are too old, too injured, or too frail to lift weights, and that strength training is only for the big muscle guys. This is a huge myth that continues to persist today. Resistance training is something that should be a part of your life *for the rest of your life.* And you are never too old. In fact, a 2013 study in the *Journal of Clinical Interventions in Aging* revealed that resistance training twice a week over the course of two months considerably improved mobility and muscle strength in people seventy-seven to ninety-seven years of age. Ninety-seven! And with increased mobility and muscle strength, all your daily activities become easier.

Francine started on a program that used prescriptive exercises to rebuild the parts of her body that were weak and to place weight on certain joints to help with bone density. She no longer needed a cane or feared for her safety during basic movements, and she understood the essential exercises she needed to do weekly to keep her body strong. She was able to return to all her daily activities and even took up golf with her husband—a sport she avoided previously because she could not walk the course and feared the swinging motion would hurt her back.

Fact: Osteoporosis and osteopenia-related fractures are most common in the spine, hips, and wrist. Weight-bearing exercises and resistance training have been shown to increase bone density and prevent fractures.

The Strong Benefits of Strength Training

Resistance training was once only the domain of men who competed in such sports as football and rugby or possessed a naturally muscular frame. The average person saw very little need to engage in weight training. And to this day women avoid it because of the negative stereotype that resistance training will make them big and bulky. If you are injured, you no doubt are fearful to walk into a gym where people are grunting and grimacing as they exercise. You probably think resistance training is not for you and could cause further injury and harm. These old concepts have become folklore for many. In the new world, resistance training is something that everyone can and *should* participate in—whether you have a fracture, arthritis, an autoimmune disease, or fibromyalgia. The truth is, you can't get out of persistent pain *without* movement.

Strength training not only helps you burn fat—and therefore lose more weight—but also has numerous health benefits. It reduces and reverses the muscle loss associated with sarcopenia and improves your physical function. It builds tissue and muscle mass, and you obtain better benefits in a shorter period of time. It's much more efficient than cardio or endurance training, which actually breaks down your tissue (more on this later). Strength training truly is your key to better health, less pain, and real weight loss.

Ten Myths of Resistance Training

- I'm too old.
- I'm too injured.
- I have a disease.
- It's not good for women.
- My muscles will get tight.
- I will get bulky like Arnold Schwarzenegger or the Hulk!
- Only men benefit from weight training.
- I won't burn enough calories—I need cardio!
- It will hurt and increase my pain.
- I need something low impact.

Reversing Muscle Loss

As we have become sedentary and heart disease has emerged as the leading cause of death, regular exercise has been promoted as the means to a desirable body weight. More attention and emphasis has been focused on the problem of sarcopenia (age-related muscle loss), shining a spotlight on resistance training—and with good reason. Basically, when you lose muscle, it slows down your metabolism and packs on the pounds. Clinically, those with age-related muscle loss will see earlier and more rapid bone loss, metabolic decline, fat gain, pain, diabetes, and metabolic syndrome.

It is never too late to rebuild your muscle, regardless of your condition. Many studies have shown that brief sessions of regular resistance training two to three times per week can increase muscle mass. In fact, this has been proven even up to the tenth decade of life—that's one hundred years of age! A study with more than 1,600 subjects between the ages of twenty-one and eighty revealed that after ten weeks of resistance training, participants had a lean weight increase of up to 3 pounds. Now, I know you want to lose weight not gain it, but 3 pounds of lean mass or muscle is what you *do* want. The benefit of strength training is that it replaces fat with lean muscle mass. The more muscle you have on your body, the higher your resting metabolism will be. This means that you will burn more calories—and thus more fat—at rest. So, even after you finish your workout, your body will continue to burn calories without you having to do anything.

Greater muscle mass uses more energy at rest for ongoing tissue maintenance. When you weight train with progressively heavier weights, it causes your body to use large amounts of energy for muscle remodeling and rebuilding that often persists for up to two days after your workout. Putting on muscle mass is one of the best things you can do to increase your metabolism. Plus, with a little more muscle mass, you look firmer and leaner. Resistance can also help improve insulin sensitivity, which helps decrease inflammation and burn fat.

Reducing Fat

Increasing your metabolic rate is a major factor in fat loss. Excessive body fat is associated with risk factors, such as increased blood sugar, cholesterol, and blood pressure, all of which contribute to the development of type 2 diabetes. Resistance training can decrease the abdominal fat tissue, increase metabolic rate, improve insulin sensitivity, and decrease abdominal fat stores. Furthermore, as you age there is a natural tendency toward insulin resistance and thus the prevalence of type 2 diabetes. Resistance training can decrease insulin resistance, improve glycemic control, and reduce abdominal fat, which is of critical importance in diabetes prevention. Resistance training can also lower hemoglobin A1c levels in diabetics, a common biomarker for blood glucose and an indicator of inflammation.

Improving Physical Function

A loss of muscle mass is accompanied by a loss of physical function, which often hinders your independence and can be one of the most frustrating aspects of pain and weight gain. If you have found it more difficult to perform some of your most basic daily activities, or you are fatigued after them, no doubt the loss of muscle mass is making daily life more difficult. People often notice that walking, stairs, and lifting become problematic. Resistance training can help reverse the effects of muscle loss related to aging, even in the elderly. In studies conducted in nursing homes, resistance training has been proven to enhance patients' movement, balance, walking speed, and a variety of common daily activities. In one study, where the average age of the subjects was eighty-nine years old, after fourteen weeks overall strength increased by 60 percent and functional independence improved by 14 percent.

If you don't want to lose your physical independence, resistance training should be a part of your weekly routine. And if you have ever needed physical therapy to recover from an injury or condition, you probably noticed that a large part of your recovery was related to getting stronger. One of the first tasks a physical therapist will perform when evaluating for an injury or disease is to look at your movement and test your muscles to assess for specific muscle groups that are weak. The only prescription for a weak muscle is to strengthen it with resistance training.

Why Strength Training Is Better than Cardio

If you have a regular routine of cardiovascular exercise, that's great! You are doing more than many people to keep yourself active. One of the most common questions I receive when someone wants to begin an exercise program is, "How much cardio do I have to do?" Certainly, doing some type of exercise that increases your heart rate has proven cardiovascular benefits. The challenge is that cardio has been so ingrained in our head, especially with regard to weight loss, that most people think there is no other option. I find this to be true of people with persistent pain, too, because they are told that the endorphins released during cardiovascular exercise have an analgesic effect, also known as the "runner's high." A runner's high certainly feels good and accessing your brain's own natural opioid pharmacy is awesome; however, you can achieve a greater level of quicker endorphin response in less time with strength training, especially burst style high-intensity interval training, which we'll discuss in more detail later in the chapter. Doesn't that sound good? *Less exercise equals more benefit.*

The other challenge with cardiovascular exercise is that quite often, especially if this is your only form of exercise, it can become repetitive. Repetitive movement works the same muscles over and over and lacks variety, which often leads to overuse injuries. Most people will find one type of exercise, such as running or cycling, and only engage in this single activity. Cycling is low impact but you are sitting, and most of you do not need to sit more. Running, despite its proclaimed health benefits, commonly causes joint pain, tendonitis, and stress fractures.

Even though aerobic exercise has cardiovascular benefits, it fails to build muscle mass and counteract sarcopenia. A 2015 study in the *Journal of Gerontology* found resistance training to be far superior to aerobic exercise with regard to building muscle. For many people, chronic and prolonged aerobic exercise can actually send the complete opposite signal, which leads to decreased strength and muscle atrophy. For someone who struggles with persistent low-grade inflammation and poor mitochondrial health, frequent cardiovascular exercise can lead to fatigue and pain.

Many people are sedentary, sit all day long, and are losing muscle mass in addition to the poor diet they are eating. It is extremely difficult to "burn off" years of a poor diet when you lack the muscle mass—even if you run upward of five hours per week. This can become a vicious cycle for many and one where you ultimately become injured. And, once you are injured, do you know what your doctor of physical therapy is going to recommend for your healing? Strengthening the muscles or groups of muscles that are weak or overused from the repetitive nature of endurance training. Remember, you are learning the most optimal way to heal, not the fastest way to injure yourself.

Learn to incorporate some daily movement into your life and you won't have to spend hours on the treadmill or running around the high school track. Purchase a pedometer to keep track of your daily movement. Aim for a minimum of 5,000 steps, preferably 8,000, and ideally 10,000. It is much more efficient and helpful for your metabolism to engage in movement throughout the day versus one large time chunk of thirty to sixty minutes doing cardio. Incorporating daily movement can be easy. Take the dog for a walk, take a walk after dinner instead of watching the negative news, and park your car a bit farther from the door to your office, home, or shopping center. Learning to include some daily movement at work is vitally important as well. A few times a day, and especially at lunch, walk or take a few flights of stairs. Adding regular movement into your life is easier and offers more of a benefit than squeezing long hours on the treadmill into your busy schedule.

Strength Training Rebuilds Muscle; Endurance Training Breaks Down Muscle

Your body is going through a constant process of break down and rejuvenation. Old cells are replaced with new ones that form to make new tissues and organs. With the right nutrition, you will rebuild and rejuvenate more than you will break down. In science this is known as anabolic (to build up) and catabolic (to break down). You can live a life where you are mostly in an anabolic state by understanding what exactly sends the signals to your body to begin the cascade of genes, hormones, and peptide messengers responsible for the rebuilding process.

The metabolic capacity of your muscle is responsible for your metabolism and the slide toward obesity, and pain. Muscle breakdown is a major factor to the contribution of the aforementioned epidemics of sedentary disease.

Endurance exercise, often referred to as cardiovascular, is catabolic; it breaks down your muscle tissue instead of rebuilding it. The reason it breaks down your tissue is that you need it for energy, since it requires you to sustain long periods of exhausting, often repetitive, exercise, such as running or cycling. Because of its repetitive nature, the stress it places on one set of muscles can also lead to inflammation, which, as you now know, leads to pain.

Strength Training Rejuvenates Your Fast Muscle Fibers

Muscles are able to move because they receive a message from your brain. Your first thought of the day—to reach and shut off the alarm clock—causes an impulse to travel from your brain, down a nerve, and to terminate in what is called the neuromuscular junction, where muscle and nerve meet. Because your body is so smart, you don't just have one type of muscle fiber. Each of us has a mix of slow muscle fiber types and fast muscle fiber types. Sarcopenia can involve the breakdown of both types of muscle, but the most detrimental and crucial to your health is the faster muscle types. Fast muscle fiber types are more prone to loss due to an injury, disease, a sedentary lifestyle, and free radicals and oxidative stress.

The fast muscle fibers are predominantly the type that you use for daily activities that require power, strength, and speed, so you want to keep and improve upon your fast muscle fibers. Even though we are born with a certain amount of both slow and fast muscle fibers, your body is incredibly adept at creating new fast muscle fibers, if given the right type of exercise. And I will give you a hint: Endurance training does not prevent the loss of or rejuvenate fast type muscle fibers. To protect and grow your fast muscle fibers, you need to engage in strength training.

The Ultimate Muscle Rejuvenation Prescription

- Incorporate short, intense exercise into your life two times per week.
- Follow the Healing Pain Program of quality protein, healthy fat, and low-glycemic meals.
- Replace endurance training with resistance training.
- Begin the day with a healing protein shake (see Appendix A).

Healing Hormones

No injections, patches, or creams are needed here. It should be no surprise that exercise benefits a variety of hormones, and these hormones are in turn responsible for building muscle, strengthening bones and tendons, healing injury, and even making you feel good. Essentially, your hormones can help with both pain management and weight loss. Some of the hormones include growth hormone, insulin-like growth factor 1 (IGF-1), and brain-derived neurotrophic factor (BDNF). Let's take a look at some of the hormonal benefits achieved from proper exercise.

The main targets for growth hormone are skeletal muscle, bone, immune cells, and fat cells. Growth hormone works to rebuild and repair muscle tissue, increase fat breakdown, stimulate cartilage and collagen for strong joints, and decrease storing sugar as fat. All of these functions result in optimal conditions in your body to promote tissue repair and recover from exercise. You can increase the secretion of this hormone with resistance and high-intensity exercise, low carbohydrate intake, intermittent fasting, and sleep. Sleep is especially critical, as a large majority of growth hormone is released while sleeping. Make sure to get at least seven to nine hours of sleep each night. And, remember, if you are beginning an exercise program, you may need a bit more, because your body is in the repair and recover mode, rebuilding a leaner, fitter, and pain-free you!

Insulin-like growth factor 1 (IGF-1) is growth hormone's right-hand man in the daily process of rebuilding a leaner and stronger you! Eight to twelve hours after growth hormone is released, IGF comes in to assist with the rebuilding and repair process. IGF has specific anabolic or growth activity. We are learning more, but it is likely that IGF is released when fat cells are destroyed and resistance exercise initiated.

Exercise increases brain-derived neurotrophic factor (BDNF) and helps preserve nerve and brain function. BDNF aids in nerve growth, reduces neurodegeneration, improves how nerves connect and transmit signals, and helps repair damaged cells in the central nervous system. It makes all the wiring in your nervous system more efficient and fluid.

We all need some brain-derived neurotrophic factor production, and exercise is one major way to get this hormone working for us. Nutrition, exercise, and mind-training techniques create the perfect trifecta to keep your BDNF flowing. Preventing degeneration of your most important organ—your brain—should be high on your list.

Sleep Away Your Pain

In 2012, a study in the *Journal of Arthritis and Rheumatism* found those with disrupted sleep patterns are more likely to develop chronic pain symptoms and struggle with weight. A solid night's sleep helps normalize stress hormones *and* releases growth hormones to help heal and repair muscle and connective tissue.

Your Brain's Natural Opioids

Your brain produces its own natural opioid chemicals that work to dampen and alleviate pain. They also have the effect of improving mood via serotonin pathways—similar to most prescription antidepressant drugs. And if you have an autoimmune condition, opioids activate special immune cells called Tregs (regulatory T cells), which improve self-tolerance; with improved self-tolerance, there is an improvement in autoimmune symptoms. Tregs prevent the body from "attacking itself."

In the peripheral nervous system (outside your brain), beta-endorphins produce analgesia and exert opioid-like effects. Specifically, they prevent substance P, a key protein involved in the transmission of pain. In the central nervous system (brain), beta-endorphins work similarly; however, instead of inhibiting substance P, they exert their analgesic effect by inhibiting the release of GABA, an inhibitory neurotransmitter, resulting in excess production of dopamine. Dopamine is associated with pleasure.

The opioids that occur naturally within our body seem likely to be assigned a significant role in the integrated hormonal and metabolic response to exercise. Most studies have demonstrated that serum concentrations of endogenous opioids (beta-endorphins) increase in response to exercise. Elevated serum beta-endorphin concentrations induced by exercise have been linked to several psychological and physiological changes, including positive mood state changes, feelings of euphoria, and altered pain perception. There are lots of reasons here to get moving and feel good!

Resistance Training Guidelines and Exercises

A resistance or strength-training program should be performed a minimum of two days per week, with at least 24 hours of rest in between sessions. If you have never done any type of strength training, or you are older or frail, begin with lighter weight that you can comfortably lift for two sets of 12 to 15 repetitions. As you gain strength, you will increase the weight and decrease the repetitions. For healthy adults, choose a weight you can comfortably lift for 8 to 12 repetitions and two sets with good form and moderate exertion.

You may not know which exercises you should be doing, since the gym has so many options. I understand your frustration and will provide guidance on the best strength-training movements for improving your pain and weight loss. There are five types of exercises you should aim to incorporate: pushing, pulling, squatting, lunging, and core. These are the five basic movements you need, and from here you will begin to branch out and enjoy all the variations.

You will notice that these are compound and functional movements. This means that you are moving more than one joint at a time and performing exercises that mimic daily activities. For example, the simple squat-type exercise is used every day in daily life to lift or pick something up, and it involves the muscles of your lower back, hips, thighs, and lower legs, all in one movement! I prefer that you perform compound functional movements versus single-joint exercises.

Here are some other tips:

- Perform resistance training two to three times a week.
- Lift the heaviest weight you can handle with good form and minimal discomfort.

- If you are a beginner, start with a weight where you can perform between 12 and 15 repetitions. As you increase strength, increase the weight but decrease the repetitions to between 8 and 12 repetitions.
- You can split up your resistance training with pushing and squatting on one day and pulling and lunges on another. Core can be performed on both days.
- In the beginning you can allow for 90 seconds of rest between each set, but as you progress only allow for 60 seconds.
- If you are frail or elderly, you may choose to perform one set the first two weeks. After that aim for two to three sets of each exercise, with 8 to 10 repetitions in each set.
- Resistance training never gets easier! If you find your workouts becoming routine and easy, increase the weight.

Moderate muscle soreness is normal after a workout. This soreness is felt in the meaty part of a muscle, such as the middle part of your thigh. This soreness is your body rebuilding healthy muscle—hooray! If you experience pain along a tendon or joint line—such as the inside of your knee—this is not good, and you may be performing the exercise incorrectly. Check your form, decrease the weight, or enlist the help of a physical therapist or other exercise professional. Stretching after a workout can also help to alleviate muscle tightness and maintain joint mobility. For additional instruction on exercise, visit www.drjoetatta.com/exercise.

High-Intensity Interval Training (HIIT)

HIIT is where the real magic takes place in your body. Once you are comfortable with strength training exercises, you can begin high-intensity interval training, which will enable you to step up your game and become a fat-burning machine. The best part is that you don't have to do it for an hour but only somewhere between 4 and 20 minutes. HIIT, which is also known as burst training, involves short, intense 20- to 60-second bursts of activity, with a recovery period of 30 seconds to one minute. You should aim for 4 to 12 total minutes of high intensity bursts and eventually work up to a twenty-minute workout. It should feel intense, and you should be breathless by the end of the workout. When my clients whose exercise program has lacked intensity make this one change, they often see fat-burning results within two weeks.

High-intensity interval training also has a positive impact on your blood sugar levels, improves insulin sensitivity, and can help reverse metabolic syndrome. A 2015 study in the *Journal of Diabetes Research* found that patients with diabetes preferred HIIT over long-duration cardiovascular exercise. HIIT burns the most fat in the shortest amount of time, and your body will continue to burn calories for up to forty-eight hours following a workout. It also reduces your risk of cardiovascular disease, decreases blood pressure, enhances your immunity, and increases brain-derived neurotrophic factor (BDNF), preventing neurodegeneration.

Once you begin high-intensity interval training, it's important to remember that you still need to be careful. Some people begin to overtrain their body, but the higher the intensity of exercise, the more cautious you should be about rest and recovery. HIIT raises your heart rate above 70 percent, but it shouldn't make it impossible for you to move normally the next day. Just as with resistance or strength training, you should also rest for one day between HIIT workouts.

Intense and Intelligent Exercise

Now that you understand how your muscles work, let's talk about how to activate the faster muscle fibers so you can effectively lose weight. This is exciting for me, as I have spent years not only teaching this to my clients in an effort to help with weight loss and injury prevention but also, to this day, I still see many people spending day after day and hour after hour on the bike, treadmill, or running. Again, some exercise is better than no exercise, but I have always been interested in the fastest and most efficient way to lose fat and get in shape.

The best part and what people love most about HIIT is that it takes minimal time—benefits can be seen with as little as seven minutes! And once you get into it, you will find you need no more than twenty minutes three times a week. With all this newfound time, you can devote yourself to preparing some delicious Healing Pain Diet Recipes!

HIIT always involves alternating short intervals of high intensity exercise with short intervals of rest in between. The intensity is the key—to create the changes needed to blast fat and grow mitochondria, you need to be working at a certain level of intensity. The other positive attribute is that HIIT training involves rotating through many different types of exercise or intervals. An effective HIIT workout will involve a variety of exercises with the goal to stimulate as many muscle groups as possible. And with a variety of exercise comes the added benefit of improvements in strength, flexibility, endurance, balance, and coordination. All of this change feeds your brain and releases growth hormone and BDNF. It improves the plasticity of your nervous and musculoskeletal system. Your thirty minutes of steady cardio on the treadmill or stationary bike in no way has the combined effects of HIIT.

In one session of HIIT not only will you burn fat and calories while you are working out, but you will also continue to have the increased metabolic effects for up to forty-eight hours following your workout. HIIT is known for having this "afterburn" effect. This is attributed to your mitochondria's need for oxygen after a high intensity workout. Because of this, after you complete your workout, your oxygen consumption and calorie burning remain elevated for up to forty-eight

Exercise Intensity Table

Intensity Level	Heart Rate	Physical Signs and Clues
Light	40–55 percent	Barely noticeable increase in breathing and no sweating
Moderate	55–69 percent	Breathing becomes deeper and faster; you can still talk but only in short sentences; sweating will be noticed after 10 minutes.
High	70 percent +	Breathing is deep and rapid; it's difficult to carry on a conversation; sweating begins within 3 to 5 minutes.

hours. This higher metabolic level continues as your muscle cells are repaired and restored. Your body will burn fat and use it as fuel and nutrients for recovery. Lower and moderately intense exercise does not have an afterburn effect and only works while you are doing it. HIIT continues to burn fat even when you are not moving!

Weight Loss, Not Muscle Loss

If you have ever started a program for weight loss before and noticed that you were losing weight but also getting flabby at the same time, there is a good reason. It can be hard not to lose muscle mass along with fat. The reason for this is that many fad diet programs are nutritionally imbalanced, are void of essential nutrients, overly restrict calories, and recommend doing cardio for many days and hours. Being nutrient deficient completely robs your body and leaves it no choice but to begin to break down its own muscle tissue in an effort to supply nutrients, such as protein. This places your body in a stressed state and, combined with the catabolic effects of increased endurance exercise on an already taxed system, we have a recipe for enhancing sarcopenia. Your body is starving and stressed.

By following the Healing Pain Diet combined with HIIT, you will preserve and build your lean muscle mass while blasting fat and serving your body with the essential nutrients it needs to thrive. HIIT, along with the other key concepts of the Healing Pain Program, work to enhance growth hormone responsible for fat loss and lean muscle gains.

HIIT Burns Belly Fat and Controls Appetite

Your belly fat is what you most want to burn off, because it is responsible for inflammation and your pain! A study published in the *American Journal of Physical Medicine & Rehabilitation* cited sixty-two overweight and obese subjects who performed HIIT with strength training two to three times per week over the course of nine months and saw significant improvement in both waist circumference measurements and overall body fat. In contrast, longer exercise sessions exceeding one hour stimulated overproduction of stress hormones, such as cortisol, which contributes to the storage of abdominal fat.

In a study on the effects of HIIT on fat loss, Australian researchers cited a lower perceived appetite after HIIT training. Researchers suggest this is due to release of the satiety hormone called peptide YY, as well as lowered levels of the appetite stimulating hormone ghrelin, after high intensity work. And the evidence gets even better because HIIT works best when paired with a resistance training program. Sound familiar? Studies suggest that strength training has also been proven to release hormones that regulate appetite during and after exercise.

You Have to Start Somewhere

It can be difficult to begin an exercise program if you have been overweight and in pain or have an arthritic disease. You are not the person who is going to start working out four times a week for an hour. But if you can commit to just five minutes of HIIT three times a week, you will see that the opioid-like endorphin effects that modulate pain and elevate your mood, as well as the benefits of growth hormone to burn fat, are well worth it. There is not a remedy or pill that can have the same variety of profound and lasting effects on the body as exercise.

In a 2015 study in the *Journal of Applied Physiology*, women with rheumatoid arthritis performed HIIT, consisting of four-minute intervals twice a week for ten weeks on a stationary upright bike. HIIT resulted in significant improvements in BMI, body fat, and waist circumference, which all decreased, while muscle mass increased. Furthermore, HIIT decreased C-reactive protein (a measure of inflammation) coupled with changes in disease activity and pain.

Think you are too old, injured, or have a disease that will prevent you from exercising intensely? HIIT has been studied in all types of conditions from obesity to diabetes, cardiovascular disease, and even autoimmune conditions. In 2015, a study in the medical journal *PLOS ONE* found that high intensity cardiovascular exercise combined with resistance training was safe, well tolerated, and improved muscle strength and endurance in patients with multiple sclerosis.

How Do I Know if I'm Working "Intensely" Enough?

The key with HIIT is to reach a high enough intensity to raise your heart rate to a certain threshold. Remember, HIIT only lasts seconds, but the intensity in those moments is critical. An easy way to measure your intensity is on a simple 1 to 10 scale, with 1 being super easy and 10 being maximum. On a scale of 1 to 10, you need to be at a 7 or greater to achieve the physiologic benefit of HIIT. The intensity is what accelerates fat loss and improves mitochondrial health and releases opioid endorphins to modulate pain. For quick, five-minute beginner HIIT programs, visit www.drjoetatta.com/HIIT.

Beginner Program

Beginner 1	Exercise	Work	Rest	Total Time	5 Minutes
	Marching in Place	:20	:10		
	Sit to Stand	:20	:10		
	Wall Pushups	:20	:10		
	Modified Plank	:20	:10		
	Repeat Twice	Rest 30 Seconds			

Beginner 2	Exercise	Work	Rest	Total Time	5 Minutes
	Marching in Place	:20	:10		
	Mini-squats	:20	:10		
	Wall Pushups	:20	:10		
	Pelvic Lifts	:20	:10		
	Repeat Twice	Rest 30 Seconds			

Intermediate HIIT Program

Intermediate 1	Exercise	Work	Rest	Total Time	7 minutes
	Squats	:30	–		
	Kneeling Pushups	:30	–		
	Lunges	:30	–		
	Planks	:30	–		
	Repeat Three Times	30 Second Rest			

Intermediate 2	Exercise	Work	Rest	Total Time	7 minutes
	Jumping Jacks	:30	–		
	Tricep Dips	:30	–		
	Reverse Lunges	:30	–		
	Planks	:30	–		
	Repeat Three Times	30 Second Rest			

continues

continued

Advanced HIIT Program

Advanced 1	Exercise	Work	Rest	Total Time	10 Minutes
	Squats	1 minute	–		
	Push ups	1 minute	–		
	Lunges	1 minute	–		
	Bicycle	1 minute	–		
	Repeat Twice	1 minute rest			

Advanced 2	Exercise	Work	Rest	Total Time	15 Minutes
	Squats	1 minute	–		
	Pushups	1 minute	–		
	Lunges	1 minute	–		
	Planks	1 minute	–		
	Repeat Three Times	1 minute Rest			

HIIT with Resistance

Program 1	Exercise	Work	Rest	Total Time	15 Minutes
	Squats With Shoulder Press	1 minute	–		
	Lunges With Bicep Curls	1 minute	–		
	Bent Over Rows	1 minute	–		
	Bicycle	1 minute	–		
	Repeat Three Times	1 minute Rest			

Program 2	Exercise	Work	Rest	Total Time	15 Minutes
	Lateral Lunge With Shoulder Press	1 minute	–		
	Reverse Lunge With Bicep Curls	1 minute	–		
	Kettle Bell Swings	1 minute	–		
	Chops With Medicine Ball	1 minute	–		
	Repeat Three Times	1 minute Rest			

Combining the Healing Pain Diet with strength training and HIIT, you have a great program for lowering inflammation, which will make you feel much better. If you have been following the Healing Pain Movement Program, you now realize that moving your body—even a body that has been in pain for a long time—is actually good for you and helps you feel much better. You are beginning to reverse muscle loss, reduce fat, and improve your daily physical function. All of this exercise is stimulating the hormones that are responsible for building your muscles and improving nerve function. You should definitely be noticing some significant weight loss by now, especially around your abdomen, and feeling a marked alleviation in your pain. If you find that you are having trouble with the exercise portion of the Healing Pain Program because you are still fearful of movement, the next chapter will help you overcome your fear with some simple techniques to reset your brain in pain.

Dr. Joe's Pain Relief Reminders

- Movement is essential to alleviate persistent pain.
- Strength training reverses muscle loss (sarcopenia), reduces fat, and improves physical function.
- Begin strength or resistance training for a minimum of two days per week, focusing on the following five types of exercise: pushing, pulling, squatting, lunging, and core.
- High-intensity interval training (HIIT) requires minimal time for maximum fat burn.
- HIIT can create changes in just seven minutes that would take more than an hour with steady endurance training.

Part IV

The Healing Pain Mind Program

10

USE YOUR BRAIN, STOP YOUR PAIN

Do you want to know the fastest way to stop your pain? You already know it's not a pill, potion, lotion, or injection. You have read a lot about nutrition, movement, and exercise and their influence on your pain; implement all of the information you have absorbed from the previous chapters. The truth is that despite what you have been told, pain is created in your *brain*—and nowhere else! Not in your joints, not in your muscles, only in your brain. Understanding how pain works in your brain and what you can do about it may be the secret to the speediest form of recovery. It will skyrocket your ability to heal your pain now, and if you have struggled for years with persistent (chronic) pain, this knowledge has been the missing link in your recovery—the one important link that no one has explained. Uncovering some simple lessons about your brain will ultimately help you conquer your pain. Along with the other tools I provided in this book, you will now have everything you need to end your persistent pain and remove the label "chronic" from your life.

The good news is that you have the power to change to your benefit the information your brain receives. The first step is awareness, and once you acknowledge the fact that all of these factors influence your brain, you can learn effective coping strategies for overcoming the negative thoughts, emotions, behaviors, memories, and sensations, so that you can positively influence your brain to refocus on healing your pain.

Use Your Brain to Treat Your Pain

Now it is time to take back your brain and leverage that wonderful state called plasticity to cure your pain. How do we know pain really exists in the brain? People who have lost an arm or a leg often complain of an experience known as phantom limb pain. This is when they experience pain as if the limb were still present. These feelings are completely real and often worsen during stress. Phantom limb pain reveals that even though a limb is absent, the brain still recognizes it as present. I like to think of this as a GPS in your brain that represents your body. Inside your brain is a representation of your entire body called the homunculus, which is a virtual map in your brain of your body.

The more receptors there are in a given area of skin, the larger that area's map will be represented on the surface of the brain. As a result, the size of each body region in the homunculus is related to the density of sensory receptors on your skin's surface. The face, lips, and hands take up a lot of real estate, because they have numerous sensory nerve endings for touch. Studies show that with phantom limb pain, changes occur in the brain (plasticity) in this virtual body. For example, if your foot was amputated, we might see that the area in your brain that occupied your foot is less distinct and now has overlap with your hip. Scientists call this smudging, and it refers to a loss of distinct boundaries for body parts in your brain. This is how foot pain can be mistaken for hip pain, and shoulder pain can be mistaken for hand pain. So, quite simply, your brain gets confused between which body part is which, and right and left sides also become confused. It can even mistake a part of your body as moving when it actually isn't! All of this confusion inside your brain is going on without you even knowing it, although this should start to connect some of the dots for you when it comes to your persistent pain or another weird indescribable pain you may have.

Move in Your Brain First

You already know how important movement is for alleviating your pain, and I am sure this is not the first time you have heard that. But let's be honest, when you fear movement due to pain, you don't feel much like exercising. Well, I have good news for you! You can actually trick your brain into thinking it is moving or exercising and in return lower your sensitivity to pain. As you lower your sensitivity, you can then begin to exercise for real—safely and comfortably. This brain training technique is called graded motor imagery or simply motor imagery. It is a type of rehabilitation program used to treat the most persistent pain and movement problems. Graded motor imagery is broken down into three unique stages, with techniques that exercise your brain in a different way. The three stages of graded motor imagery are:

1. **Left-right discrimination**—The ability to identify a body part as left or right. For example, if your left hand has been in chronic pain for a long time, it can be difficult to distinguish between which hand is left or right. This is often unnoticeable to the average person.

2. **Explicit motor imagery**—Watching or imagining a body part in a specific motion or position. This is accomplished by thinking about a body part moving, without actually moving. Imagined movements can actually be hard work if you are in pain. By imagining movements, you use similar brain areas as you would when you actually move. You have seen athletes, such as gymnasts, practice motor imagery before a competition or routine. This also explains why you can watch an action movie or sports game and feel tired afterward. You are moving in your brain.

3. **Mirror therapy**—If you were to put your left hand behind a mirror and right hand in front, you can trick your brain into believing the reflection of your right hand in the mirror is your left. You are now exercising your left hand in your brain, particularly if you start to move your right hand. It is sort of an optical illusion, but your brain does not know the difference. Your brain is tricked into thinking the painful side is moving.

How does motor imagery work exactly? Well, in your brain there are mirror neurons, and these neurons actually fire or are active when you observe or imagine movement. Graded motor imagery has been shown to offer relief from pain and disability in some of the most difficult pain states to treat, including complex regional pain syndrome, neuropathic, carpal tunnel syndrome, and even osteoarthritis. The key with graded motor imagery is just that, it has to be graded, which means progressively increasing the intensity and duration. Just as exercise is graded, adding a few more pounds of weight each week, graded imagery is progressive. If you are imagining an activity, such as bouncing a basketball, when you can't even tap your finger on the table, it may cause pain. A 2008 study in the *Journal of Arthritis Care & Research* found that if participants engaged in motor imagery exercises that caused fear or anxiety, due to their difficulty, it actually caused the limb not only to be more painful but also to begin swelling! This is why sometimes it even hurts if you think about certain movements or see someone else move in a way that your brain finds threatening. Isn't the brain truly amazing in the way it can have an effect on the body?

Graded motor imagery can be difficult to describe in a book, so I have included some free video training that you can access at www.drjoe tatta.com/motorimagery. There are free training videos, covering all three techniques.

Pacing, Movement, and Graded Motor Imagery

Quite often, particular activities are challenging, painful, and sometimes avoided for fear of causing harm. With your new knowledge of pain (knowing that hurt does not equal harm), you can begin to move and will be able to reengage with activity. Your daily activities, exercise, and graded motor imagery should be paced—meaning you set a baseline and then progressively and steadily work toward your goal. This entails establishing a baseline for an activity; in other words, the degree to which you can participate in an activity without flaring up your pain in such a way that it can take hours or days to settle back down. This is known as a graded exposure approach to treatment. A randomized control trial in 2008 in the *Journal of Pain* found graded exposure was an effective treatment for fear in patients with chronic back pain. Just doing a bit more each day can retrain the fear out of your brain and promote flexibility with how you approach movement and pain.

How to Find Your Baseline

Your baseline is the amount of activity you can do today and know that pain won't flare up. Here is a sample dialogue I had with my patient Max, which will provide you with some sample questions you can ask yourself to find your baseline:

> How far can you walk before a flare-up?
> *I walked for 30 minutes this morning, but I was in pain by the end of the day and the next.*
> Okay. Can you walk for 20 minutes?
> *Yes, but I will still have pain that night.*
> Can you walk for 15 minutes without flaring up?
> *Yes, that I can do!*

For walking, Max's baseline is 15 minutes. With this information, he can plan for a bit further each day (16, 17, 18, 20 minutes). If you are feeling good, don't suddenly increase to 30 minutes; stay the course. Do not be tempted to break the progression you have created for yourself. Stick with your plan and goals and you will be rewarded! This can be done with every activity, including daily activities such as housework, weights, exercise, and even for athletes returning to their sport. Remember, your nervous system is sensitive, so a flare-up may occur. Accept this but remain committed to your pacing and goals—the reward is worth the effort.

Using Visualization to Conquer Fear

Too often patients allow their identity to become intertwined with their pain, and they only see a life filled with limitation stretching out before them, which can sabotage the road to healing. This was true of my patient Sandy. When Sandy first walked into the office, it was apparent she was someone who knew how to take care of her body.

She was a gorgeous thirty-nine-year-old ballet dancer who recently transitioned to theater dance and was in one of the hottest shows on Broadway.

Sandy had danced professionally for almost two decades and had never sustained an injury until recently, when a back injury caused her to miss a few weeks of performances. Not dancing and missing performances was crushing to her, because she had spent nearly every day of her life dancing.

Sandy's spinal X-ray had revealed a "sacralization," where two of her lower vertebrae were fused together, which occurs naturally in a small percent of the population. Most people probably don't even know they have this until they receive an X-ray. Sandy was likely born with this and had been just fine, "living and leaping" pain-free, for decades. The one thing Sandy did have now, which I wish she didn't, was a diagnosis. A body of evidence-based research reveals that discussing medical terminology, detailed anatomic descriptions, and providing a diagnosis, such as herniated disk, slipped disk, rupture, and so on, can be more crippling than the actual problem. Often this causes fear, and that fear leads to catastrophizing thoughts, which I noticed in Sandy.

I knew the diagnosis of having fused vertebrae was being interpreted by Sandy's brain as a threat. Her fears were worse than the actual pain itself—or even the reality of her condition. Her diagnosis caused fear and anxiety on a deep level about her career, ability to earn a living, identity (she had been dancing since she was three years old), and even caused her to question whether she would be able to negotiate pregnancy without becoming disabled!

I knew that a huge part of her recovery was going to involve redirecting her thoughts and intentions. She had already taken two weeks off from dancing and was not really doing much activity other than walking. It was my job to stop the pain train before she turned it into chronic pain. In addition to the graded exercise program we did together, I started Sandy on a series of visualization exercises each night that involved graded motor imagery.

I asked her to spend five to ten minutes with her eyes closed and envision herself dancing in her mind. Most dancers can remember routines they did from years ago. I instructed her to begin with simple dance moves she could do as a child—basic ballet movements she learned in her first class—and then progressively move through more difficult rehearsals and recitals she'd performed in over the years. As she grew stronger in therapy, I instructed her to deepen her visualization by lengthening the time of the exercise as well as increasing the difficulty of her dancing. In the final weeks of therapy, I encouraged her to add emotion to her exercise—to imagine a time when she felt strong, free, and happy dancing, or one where the audience gave her a standing ovation and cheered due to her beauty, strength, and grace. I was trying to recruit as many parts of her brain and mirror neurons as possible.

In six weeks Sandy's spine was not only strong but she had also repatterned the feelings of fear and anxiety out of her consciousness and replaced them with those of strength, courage, and joy. Often you need to get out of your body and back into your head for the healing to begin. It's more important to focus on the recovery than the cause. Physical pain can be a strong manifestation of your thoughts of fear, anxiety, anger, or guilt.

Always remember that you are not your diagnosis. And if you find yourself focused on worst-case scenarios, try using visualization exercises to help ease your anxiety and rechannel your energy in a more positive direction. Imagining yourself fully recovered and engaging in the activities you once did easily will have an enormous impact on your recovery and how you approach your healing and transformation.

Attack Thoughts and Pain

Above everything else, your brain's primary function is to keep you safe. From your brain's perspective, your safety comes first and foremost above all other functions. It reminds me of when I went skiing with a friend who was not wearing a ski helmet. The mountain we were skiing on required skiers to wear a helmet to be allowed to ski. When we tried to board the ski lift, the instructor prevented my friend from boarding and said, "You need to wear a helmet; skiing can be dangerous."

My friend, an expert skier, said, "I'm not a beginner. I've been skiing for years—nothing is going to happen!"

The instructor replied, "Safety never takes a holiday!"

The same dialogue is happening in your brain at all times. Your brain never takes a holiday from your safety and wants to keep you safe from danger at *all* times. The interesting aspect about your brain is that danger (and safety) can be *actual or perceived*. The actual is easy to understand—an accident, a fight, or your house on fire. The perceived can be more difficult to conceptualize, although this is what your brain deals with on a daily basis and is thwarting your efforts to live pain free. Your thoughts about actual or pending experiences can and *do* cause significant physical changes in your body that can have a profound effect on your pain. Ultimately, your brain understands and only asks two questions upon which it bases all of its actions:

- Am I being attacked?
- Am I being supported?

You can now begin thinking about your thoughts every hour and decide whether they are thoughts of attack or thoughts of support. Most of us never take inventory of our thoughts or realize that much of what we think and say enters directly into our subconscious mind and is stored.

Take a few moments every hour and begin to think about your attack thoughts first, as you will need to recognize them to fully heal. Some examples may include:

- *I've got arthritis in my back.*
- *I am diabetic.*
- *I hurt so much.*
- *I need to get in to see my doctor.*
- *I can't do X.*
- *This pain is never going to go away.*

These thoughts can signal "attack" to your brain. If your brain feels you are being attacked, it will spring into action and defend you. The production is a highly efficient and effective way for your brain to send a message to you, alerting you that you need protection. Notice that no injury has occurred, but your thoughts are the generator of your pain.

Try contrasting your attack thoughts with thoughts of support, such as:

- *I love the new recipes on my diet.*
- *I am so grateful for my (kids, wife, house).*
- *I am really enjoying learning about how to make myself healthy again.*
- *I am recovering from (diabetes, arthritis, injury).*
- *Even though I hurt today, I did 15 minutes of exercise.*

Use the following chart to make a list of your attack thoughts versus those thoughts that promote safety. Tally up your results. Do you have far more attack thoughts than safety thoughts? Your job is to tip the scales in the right direction, so that pain has a smaller chance of being a constant in your life. With fewer attack thoughts, your body will create less pain and the stress chemicals that promote the storage of fat. If you are in pain, you probably have more danger signals or one *huge* danger signal; conversely, if you are not in pain, you may have a number of safety signals or possibly one *huge* safety signal.

Signs of Attack Thoughts

1. I hope the debt collector doesn't call today.

2. This traffic jam is going to make me late.

3. I'm always fighting with my husband/wife.

4. _____

5. _____

6. _____

7. _____

8. _____

9. _____

10. _____

Signs of Safety

1. My morning workout felt great.

2. I had so much fun at dinner with my friends.

3. I'm so excited that I lost 5 pounds!

4. _____

5. _____

6. _____

7. _____

8. _____

9. _____

10. _____

False Alarms

You may also notice some false alarms, when something seemed to be a danger signal but then changes to a safety signal; for example, your test results come back negative and you now have a renewed feeling of health and vitality; the exercise you thought was too difficult starts to become easier after a few weeks; or the nutritional changes you thought made no sense or were not very palatable in the beginning now are tasty, and you notice your pants seem looser.

Forgiveness

For many of my patients who have struggled with pain and other chronic health conditions that required a major shift in their life, feelings of fear, anger, and guilt were at times repressed and at other times sitting on the surface, almost palpable to both them and me. Healing can rarely occur without forgiveness—and this includes forgiving yourself. Unforgiving emotions will continue to fester as fear, anger, and guilt. Forgiveness requires you to be willing to let go of resentment and negative judgment, toward the people or events that have offended or injured you, and instead choose compassion, generosity, and love. This is a choice requiring a deliberate internal process, but it does not mean that you must engage in reconciliation or return to a vulnerable emotional or physical state. If you are in pain or injured, you may find that forgiving others or yourself may ultimately help you feel better.

Forgiveness can be beneficial for people who have suffered accidents and injuries or who have chronic diseases that cause persistent pain. Because the need for recovery can stem from events both within our control, such as poor lifestyle choices, and those outside of our control, such as a car accident, many may be struggling with issues of blame, responsibility, anger, and resentment. Because of this, forgiveness can be an important coping mechanism. It can be especially helpful because those who demonstrate higher levels of forgiveness may have more energy available for their recovery, rather than allowing stress, anger, fear, and guilt to consume their every thought.

A 2012 study in *Disability & Rehabilitation* examined how forgiveness affected patients in an outpatient physical therapy center.

Forgiveness of self was one of the most important factors—more important than forgiving others. According to the study, those who were able to forgive themselves had higher levels of healthy behavior, resulting in better overall physical health and reduced pain. Interestingly, the study found that participants had a much harder time forgiving themselves than forgiving other people.

While forgiving yourself may be challenging, it clearly has a significant impact on your ability to heal and can improve your overall success. If you find yourself struggling with attack thoughts, anger, blame, fear, and guilt, try being more compassionate toward yourself and engaging in forgiveness as another tool for moving forward in your healing journey. Forgiveness is an emotion-focused coping strategy that can help deal with interpersonal stressors. A 2014 study in the *American Journal of Scientific Research* found forgiveness was not only effective in decreasing pain in women who struggled with fibromyalgia, but also that forgiveness was a strategy within the patients' personal control.

Those on a spiritual pathway know the importance of forgiveness. For many, forgiveness offers a sense of peace and opens up space in a mind that can be cluttered with grievances. The unforgiving mind is often angry, depressed, without calm, and unable to release pain. Negative feelings that repeatedly enter your mind are perceived as attack thoughts to your brain, and attack thoughts can signal the danger alarm for pain. Think about all the items surrounding your pain against which you might harbor negative feelings. These can be the people, places, and past experiences that are implicated in your particular neurotag of pain. Seeking help from a professional or spiritual coach can help you release these thoughts. Many people can escape their pain by giving up grievances and working toward forgiveness.

Acceptance and Commitment Therapy

Breaking the persistent cycle of chronic pain and addressing the various lifestyle changes needed can seem overwhelming, and at times it can be more of a mental challenge than a physical one (although by now you know the two are inseparable). Still, many have enlisted the

Technologies for Trauma and Resilience—
The Heart-Brain Connection

Post-traumatic stress disorder (PTSD) can result from sexual abuse, physical abuse, emotional abuse, domestic violence, childhood neglect, military combat, and experiences where someone is exposed to multiple life-threatening events. Treatment for PTSD requires a multimodal approach. Problems associated with this disorder include emotional dysregulation and loss of a sense of safety, trust, and self-worth. There is a tendency for these clients to develop persistent pain. Focusing on positive emotions, such as appreciation and gratitude, can greatly reduce the effects of stress and deliver you to a calmer, more peaceful state.

There are devices that use heart rhythm feedback to help people measure their emotional state in real time, so users can learn what works when it comes to emotion management. Such devices, when applied with emotion-refocusing techniques, allow users to manage stress and gain more control over their well-being. A few technologies like this are on the market; the emWave is the most widely used. Over ten thousand health professionals around the country use it to help patients that suffer from reoccurring stress and anxiety. Heart Math is a personalized app that helps emotional states that become overwhelming. This unique training system objectively monitors your heart rhythms and displays the physiological level of coherence—an optimal state in which the heart, mind, and emotions are operating in sync and in balance, and the immune, hormonal, and nervous systems function in a state of harmonious coordination.

help of a mental health professional to guide them to health and help them reframe pain. If I asked you what gets in the way of your having a happy and fulfilled life, you might say pain or the fear of pain. If you have lived with persistent pain, it can be easy to avoid all the activities that cause you pain, such as work, social events, practitioners, and exercise. Pain makes you move away from anything you associate with pain. Acceptance and commitment therapy (ACT) is a form of cognitive behavioral therapy guided by a mental health professional. It is a therapeutic approach that uses an acceptance and mindfulness process and a commitment and behavioral change process to produce greater psychological flexibility.

Greater psychological flexibility allows you to mindfully or consciously maintain contact with the present moment or persist with behaviors when doing so serves valued ends. This could mean sticking with your exercise program, even though you may feel some discomfort, consistently cooking healthy meals versus the ease of takeout, or not canceling appointments for therapy. The three pillars of ACT are (1) **A**ccepting instead of rejecting experiences, (2) **C**hosen instead of automatic unaware behaviors, and (3) **T**aking action instead of being acted on. Unlike traditional cognitive behavioral therapy, ACT is not focused on changing thoughts or emotions but instead is more focused on helping people develop the skills to make better choices and behaviors.

As humans, our natural tendency toward pain is to avoid that which causes it or figure out a way to eliminate it completely. Acceptance is important for those who have struggled with pain. Pain, at times, is a necessary part of human life. The lack of acceptance can lead patients to have the expectation that the only successful outcome is complete freedom from pain. There are many ways to measure functional progress, including more freedom to socialize, returning to work, increased activity or exercise, enjoying family time, better quality sleep, and a return to joyful hobbies. The commitment part of ACT changes focus from disability and limitations to abilities and coaching on ways to move toward value-based activities. ACT can be an invaluable tool to help you overcome pain avoidance behaviors and engage with those that bring value to your pain experience.

Mindful Meditation

Mindfulness-based stress reduction (MBSR) can be effective in reducing pain and emotional distress and improving function in patients with chronic pain. Meditation has been found to improve a wide spectrum of health-related outcomes. A 2004 study in the *Journal of Psychosomatic Research* found that mindfulness-based meditation practices have positive health benefits for those with chronic pain, cancer, heart disease, depression, anxiety, and generalized stress. Training in mindfulness meditation improves anxiety, depression, stress, and pain. Mindfulness-related health benefits include better control over your thoughts and emotions, positive mood, and acceptance, each of which has been associated with reducing pain.

Mindfulness has also been related to measureable decreases in stress hormones, such as cortisol. Seventy-seven patients with fibromyalgia, participating in a ten-week mindfulness meditation-based stress-reduction program, showed improvement in overall well-being, pain, sleep, fatigue, and the experience of feeling refreshed in the morning, as well as improved coping strategies and attitudes toward fibromyalgia.

In the early 1980s, clinical studies of mindfulness began with Jon Kabat-Zinn's groundbreaking work with chronic pain patients. He hypothesized that training in mindfulness would lessen pain by altering emotional responses to pain and enhancing acceptance-related coping strategies. Over the course of a five-year study, it was found that chronic pain patients who completed an eight-week MBSR program significantly improved their pain symptoms and overall quality of life, even up to four years after completion of this initial training. Measureable pain relief after four years is life changing.

In hundreds of studies conducted over the past decade, researchers have examined meditation's effects on people, such as attention regulation, awareness of the body, depression, post-traumatic stress disorder, and addiction. Scientists have also studied the use of meditation as a treatment for pain. A Wake Forest University study revealed an approximately 40 percent reduction in pain intensity ratings during meditation. This study took fifteen healthy volunteers and performed MRI scans of their brain while inducing pain. In the four days that followed, a certified instructor taught the subjects mindfulness meditation (to focus on a sense, often his or her breath, while accepting transient thoughts). On the fifth day, the researchers scanned the volunteers again, once while not meditating, and another time while meditating, with pain induced during both sessions. The study discovered that by activating and reinforcing some areas of the brain used in pain processing, meditation has the overall effect of helping to reduce pain intensity in patients. Other theories exist on how meditation helps pain, including that it decreases stress, which in turn decreases pain.

The 5-Minute Mantra Meditation

As a beginner, I recommend starting with this type of meditation because it is short and simple. Repeating a mantra or word is all that is required for this to induce relaxation. Suggested words include *release, relax, peace, silence, love,* or any other expression of positivity, vitality, or relaxation that works for you. Sit comfortably in a chair or semireclined in a quiet place. You should not be lying down, because you do not want to fall asleep. Close your eyes and take a few deep breaths. Begin repeating your one-word mantra slowly but repeatedly in your mind for five minutes. Once complete, spend a minute in silence. You can do this exercise in the middle of a busy day and as an effective means to decrease stress-related pain.

A Muse for Meditation

A wandering mind is not a pain-free mind. Sitting to begin a meditation practice can be a challenge when pain occupies your thoughts. Research has shown using an app can assist those who have problems meditating and starting with just three to five minutes can dramatically help you build a meditation practice. The Muse is a personalized app offering real-time feedback that helps individuals start meditating and provides quantifiable results that motivate them to continue practicing. Muse gives you feedback about your meditation in real time by translating your brain signals into sounds, such as wind or birds, as a form of biofeedback.

15-Minute Mindful Meditation

Once you have mastered the 5-Minute Mantra Meditation, you can move onto a longer mindful meditation. Mindful meditation techniques encourage the practitioner to observe wandering thoughts as they drift through the mind. The intention is to not get involved with the thoughts or to judge them, but simply to be aware of each mental note as it arises. Through mindful meditation you begin to develop an awareness of how your thoughts and feelings tend to move in particular patterns. Over time, you can become more aware of the human tendency to quickly judge experiences as "good" or "bad" ("pleasant" or "unpleasant"). With practice you will learn to "sweep" both good and bad thoughts from your mind, leaving you in a state where your mind is not preoccupied with any thought. You are learning to slow your thoughts and eventually release all thoughts, thus clearing the mind. You can begin with five minutes of mindful meditation, ultimately working your way up to fifteen.

How Do Mindfulness-Based Stress Reduction (MBSR) Techniques Reduce Pain?

Relaxation: Relaxation and promotion of the relaxation response is an important strategy for coping with pain. Meditation is not solely a relaxation technique; however, many participants find relaxation a common benefit. Pain is not only a stressful experience, but stress also exacerbates and maintains pain. Relaxation is helpful in calming down a sensitive nervous system. Relaxation also boosts your body's natural pain modifiers, such as endogenous endorphins, the "feel-good" hormones.

Acceptance: Do you feel helpless because of your pain? Does pain hold you prisoner, or do you feel like you are locking horns with it each and every day? While completely understandable, feelings of frustration, anxiety, or depression emerge when we can't control the pain. Mindfulness is about accepting what is here right now as best we can, including pain, so that we can relax and be more accepting of what we need to do next. Research shows that people who learn how to accept their pain respond better to various treatments and have better overall pain outcomes.

Mental flexibility: Negative thoughts drive negative feelings, which can sensitize our nervous systems and increase pain. Thinking very negatively about pain, or pain catastrophizing, is a strong predictor of those destined for persistent pain. Mindfulness meditation can reduce negative thoughts, as we start to see thoughts as just "mental events" rather than truths. This can decrease the impact our thoughts have on our pain. The stories and emotions created around our pain slowly dissolve. This is especially important in overcoming the past emotional injuries or feelings of depression and anxiety.

People are still aware of the pain during mindfulness meditation, but they experience it as less unpleasant, since it does not activate as many of the brain networks related to memory, emotion, and self-referential thought. In other words, meditation trains your brain to experience pain without emotional attachment and distress.

Healing Intentions

Your healing begins with your thoughts and intentions. You must understand that thoughts are never neutral, and every thought you have exerts a positive or negative effect. Everything you experience and feel is a result of your thoughts, or the influence of someone else's thoughts affecting you. Each thought you have brings peace or war, love or fear. A neutral result is impossible, and dismissing or ignoring thoughts is futile. There are a number of ways that you can set healing intentions and shift your thoughts from negative to positive to reduce your pain.

You now know that "dis-ease" in your body can be the cause of your negative mental thoughts. This is a key piece in the puzzle needed to heal—along with your nutrition and movement. Many of us have negative patterns of thinking that contribute to our pain and where our pain is located. People often describe their pain as being "manifested" in a particular body part. But after reading Chapter 3, "Your Brain in Pain," you now understand that the pain is not in your body but an output from your brain.

Along with forgiveness, your inner thoughts can be the missing ingredient necessary to break through plateaus in order to achieve better health in your life. Thoughts we hold and words we have repeated, often without consciously being aware, have a direct effect on our health. What we choose to think and say in the present moment becomes part of our longer term memory and adds to our experiences and perceptions, especially regarding pain.

A physical symptom is quite often an outer effect or a personification of what is represented in your brain. In her book *Heal Your Body,* Louise Hay states that she learned through working with many patients "for every condition in our lives, there's a *need* for it. Otherwise, we wouldn't have it." This suggests that our thoughts and emotions, especially around our pain, have a purpose. This is a huge leap for many to take, but may shed some light on how or why your pain, weight, or other chronic conditions persist despite doing everything right. By changing your mental thought patterns that contribute to disease, such as fear, anger, and guilt, you can heal your body. The process of health involves a balance between the mind, body, and spirit. Most of us are unaware of the mental patterns that are causing us pain. Clearing fear, anger, and guilt, and working on resentment and forgiveness as mentioned earlier, is part of the journey—the other piece is your mental patterns. The best part about realizing this is that you can work on mental patterns anywhere and anytime, and it does not cost a penny!

Your inner thoughts and the words you repeatedly use have created your life and your pain. Your healing lies in generating and choosing new thoughts in the current moment and using them to replace the old ones. Take one minute three times today and stop and think about your specific thoughts in that moment. If your thoughts help to shape your life experiences and emotions, is this particular thought one you want to hold? If it is a thought of fear, anger, or guilt, how do you think this will affect your health? If you want a pain-free life, you need to have thoughts that fill you with safety, not danger. Whatever you think or verbally say will be personified somehow in your body and contribute to your pain. If you are willing to change your thoughts, they will have an impact on your life.

By changing your thought patterns, you can begin to change your brain's perception of what it is experiencing. This brings us to how certain thoughts have the ability to affect certain body parts or "diseases" in the body. For example, despite losing weight, exercising, and seeing a physical therapist, you may still be experiencing lower back pain. The exercise a physical therapist prescribed may help to alleviate your pain temporarily, but the root cause of your pain may be the negative emotions around a current work situation. Your pain cannot live if you cut out its root and dispose of it. Working on healing affirmations can help to change the conscious or unconscious thought patterns that contribute to your pain. A 2015 analysis in the *Journal of Psychology* reviewed the result from 144 experimental tests looking at the effects of self-affirmation. Researchers found that self-affirmations had a positive effect on outcomes at three key points in the process of health-behavior change: (1) acceptance, (2) intention to change, and (3) subsequent behavior.

Negative thought patterns centered on fear, anger, and guilt are often at the root of other emotions and have the most potential to cause harm. The following chart outlines some of the thoughts that trigger pain in certain areas of the body and includes healing affirmations to help eradicate those thoughts.

Problem	Triggering Thoughts	Healing Affirmation
Neck pain	Anxiety. The need to control the outcomes of every situation; feeling life is out of your control.	I am safe and trust in the process of my life. I am an active participant in my life and able to let go of the outcome.
Back pain	Financial stressors and fear of not making or losing money. Fear of failure around your career. Feeling unsupported by loved ones.	Money is my friend and employment is a path to success. I trust my life and career journey. I surround myself with supportive friends and family.
Arthritis	Emotionally broken, unresolved resentment, and anger. Negative thoughts.	I release anger from my life and choose peace and love. I choose to transform resentment into forgiveness.
Autoimmune diseases	Self-hatred or issues with body image.	I am at peace with who I am and where I am on my health journey. I love my body and myself.
Chronic pain	Feeling threatened or guilty. Seeking punishment. Repetitive anger.	I am safe and open to and accept guidance in my life. Love resides in me.
Overweight	Hidden emotions of fear, anger, or guilt.	I work to forgive others and myself. I take joy in creating a life that I love and enjoy. I am safe and protected.

Purposeful Penmanship

It has been proven repeatedly that shifting your focus to the positive can dramatically improve your happiness. The key is consistency. Journaling is one of the simplest ways that I have found to consistently ensure improving my well-being and happiness, both in terms of achievement and actual, measurable, quantifiable results. Begin the day right: When you start the day on the right note, things automatically begin to fall into place. Every day.

Cultivate gratitude: Gratitude is the opposite of depression and anxiety. It's the conscious experience of appreciating the gifts in our lives and the results are tangible. Journaling can be a powerful practice to learn to place the most important and pleasurable parts of your day first.

Practice introspection: Ending the day on the right note can be essential to a good night's sleep, eliminating negative thought loops and learning more about yourself. As we sleep, our brain has the job of moving our daily experiences into its long-term memory bank. If the last thoughts you have before bed are ones of anger, guilt, or fear, this is what your brain will file away. Instead, focus on the positive or meaningful moments in your day and set your intentions for the future. Journaling can also help you track your progress, so that you have a record of how far you've come in your healing pain journey. Changing negative thought patterns to positive ones can change your brain chemistry, decrease your pain, and set you on a path toward healing.

Sample Journal Entry

Morning: Enter two things that would make today great or that you would like to achieve.

Evening: Enter two wonderful things that happened to you today.

You can also use this space to write three words of affirmation as well.

Tapping Intentions

The emotional freedom technique (EFT) is a psychological acupressure technique recommended to optimize your emotional health. EFT is based on the same energy meridians used in traditional acupuncture to treat physical and emotional ailments for more than five thousand years, without the invasiveness of needles. Instead, simple tapping with the fingertips is used to input kinetic energy onto specific meridians on the head and chest, while either tapping about a specific problem, traumatic event, or while voicing positive affirmations.

The simplest place for many to begin is with the tapping of three positive affirmations. This combination of tapping the energy meridians and voicing positive affirmation works to clear your body's bio-energy system, thus restoring balance in your mind and body, which is essential for optimal health and healing. Choose three words prior to beginning, such as *healthy*, *active*, and *energetic* or *recovering*, *vital*, and *strong*. The three words you choose should align with your goals of returning to health.

Having a Goal Can Help You Heal

One way to further enhance a positive mind-set is to set goals for yourself. You need to believe that you can achieve these goals and focus on ways to realize them. When I have patients who are struggling with their pain and who seem to remain stuck in a negative attitude, I try to get them to focus on a particular goal that they can aim for in the future. My patient Maria is a perfect example of how successful this can be when you are struggling with fear, anger, and pain.

Maria was in a terrible accident that left her an above-the-knee amputee on one side and a below the knee amputee on the other. She was having a rough time with her recovery both physically and mentally. Maria was overweight, which was complicating the physical rehabilitation process; it can be difficult to find the right fit of a prosthesis when you have so much extra tissue. Understandably, Maria bounced from depression to anger on a daily basis.

After seeing Maria for three weeks, I was told that she was refusing all treatment. Even though Maria was tough, I had begun to pierce her armor a bit during our physical therapy sessions. She was just a year younger than me at the time, which helped build trust. I knew that before the accident Maria and her boyfriend had discussed plans to get married and could use this as the *purpose* that would help her through her pain and help increase her mobility. Instead of spending so much time focusing on getting Maria to walk, I told her I was going to teach her to dance, so that she could dance with her father, husband, and friends at her wedding.

Too often clinicians fail to really ask and listen to their patients' goals. What is that one thing that will keep them connected to the process and outcome? What truly motivates them? Maria learned to walk 150 feet with a cane and two prosthetic legs in six weeks, which was seen as a success by the rehab team. But to her, the driving *purpose* of all the pain, suffering, and work she endured was to hold on to the dream of one day dancing with her dad at her wedding.

So, what is your goal or purpose? Is there something important to you that a physical recovery will enable you to do? Really think about this and set a specific intention or goal. The more concrete and measurable your goal, the more likely it will have a serious impact on your determination and progress. Is there a future event you're hoping to attend or a vacation you'd like to take with your spouse? Do you want to be healthy enough to walk your child to school or chase after him or her on the playground? Set a timeline for yourself to achieve specific goals and focus your thoughts on the positive ways that you can move closer to those goals each day.

Learning ways to retrain and reset you brain and thought patterns is a crucial part in curing your persistent pain. Graded motor imagery can help you move in your mind first to reset painful neurotags. And negative thoughts absolutely have an effect on your body and mind and can inhibit your recovery, so do your best to overcome attack thoughts that stem from fear, anger, and guilt. Instead, embrace forgiveness and acceptance, especially with regard to yourself. If you feel your fear or anxiety taking the reins, remember that this is a natural reaction to pain but that you don't have to succumb to these emotions. Practice mindfulness meditation as a way to reduce stress and emotional distress. Use a journal to shift your brain out of the negative space you are in and instead focus on healing intentions and the positive moments in your day, cultivating gratitude and introspection. Empower yourself by creating new goals, visualizing yourself achieving them, and trusting that your persistent pain will be conquered and you can return to an active life. To learn more about graded motor imagery and the other techniques to help reset your brain, visit www.drjoetatta.com/braintraining.

Dr. Joe's Pain Relief Reminders

- Graded motor imagery retrains movement in your brain, which lowers your sensitivity to pain.
- Recognize when you are susceptible to attack thoughts and consciously reframe your thinking to thoughts of safety.
- One of the most important—and possibly most difficult—elements to your healing is forgiveness. If you can learn to forgive yourself, you will have more success in your physical therapy.
- Acceptance and Commitment Therapy can also help produce greater psychological flexibility.
- Mindfulness-based stress reduction as well as journaling, EFT tapping, and healing intentions can help you experience pain with less emotional attachment.

APPENDIX A: RECIPES

Here you'll find recipes for delicious foods to support you through the program. If you are in the gut-healing or ketogenic healing phase, look for the icons to see whether a particular recipe is right for you. **G** indicates recipes for the gut-healing phase, while **K** indicates those for ketogenic healing.

GUT-HEALING RECIPES

Beverages and Shakes

BASIC HEALING PROTEIN SHAKE

Serves 1

8 ounces unsweetened coconut milk
1 scoop protein powder (for options, visit www.store.drjoetatta.com)
½ cup frozen blueberries
1 to 2 tablespoons chia seeds or flax meal (ground flaxseeds)
Handful of kale or spinach (optional)

1. Place all the ingredients in a blender and blend on high speed until smooth.

Tips for creating the perfect protein shake:
- Coconut milk is best, or use almond, cashew, or hemp milk.
- Use a quality vegan protein powder.
- Use only low-glycemic fruit.
- Throw in some greens.
- Don't forget the fiber.

~~~~~~

This shake will provide you with all the healing nutrients you need to begin your day. Chia or flaxseeds can be replaced by fiber replacement or nut butter, such as almond. Begin with 1 teaspoon and work your way up to two to increase your fiber intake.

~~~~~~

STRAWBERRY VANILLA SHAKE

Serves 1

8 ounces unsweetened coconut or almond milk
1 scoop vegan vanilla protein powder
1 tablespoon flax meal (ground flaxseeds)
½ cup frozen strawberries
Handful of spinach

1. Place all the ingredients in a blender and blend on high speed until smooth.

CHOCOLATE AVOCADO SHAKE

G

Serves 1

8 ounces unsweetened coconut or almond milk
1 scoop vegan chocolate protein powder
1 to 2 tablespoons flax meal (ground flaxseeds) or chia seeds
½ cup frozen blackberries or blueberries
½ ripe avocado
Handful of kale

1. Place all the ingredients in a blender and blend on high speed until smooth.

MINT CHIP SHAKE

G

Serves 1

8 ounces unsweetened coconut or almond milk
1 scoop vegan chocolate protein powder
1 to 2 tablespoons chia seeds
5 to 10 fresh mint leaves, or 5 drops alcohol-free peppermint extract
1 tablespoon raw cacao nibs
Additional cacao nibs and mint leaves, for garnish

1. Place all the ingredients in a blender and blend on high speed until smooth.
2. Top with additional cacao nibs and mint leaves.

CHOCOLATE CHERRY SHAKE

Serves 1

8 ounces unsweetened coconut or almond milk
1 scoop vegan chocolate protein powder
½ cup frozen cherries
1 to 2 tablespoons flax meal (ground flaxseeds)

1. Place all the ingredients in a blender and blend on high speed until smooth.

VANILLA ALMOND ESPRESSO SHAKE

G

Serves 1

8 ounces unsweetened almond milk
1 scoop vegan vanilla protein powder
1 shot brewed espresso, or ¼ cup strong brewed coffee
1 to 2 tablespoons flax meal (ground flaxseeds)
1 tablespoon almond butter
3 drops alcohol-free almond extract
Cold water or ice cubes (for thinning; optional)

1. Place all the ingredients in a blender and blend on high speed until smooth.
2. Thin with additional cold water or ice cubes, if desired.

GREEN TEA PROTEIN SHAKE

Ⓖ

Serves 1

4 ounces brewed green tea
4 ounces unsweetened coconut milk
1 scoop vegan chocolate protein powder
½ cup frozen berries
Handful of spinach or kale
1 teaspoon ground cinnamon
1 teaspoon ground ginger
Cold water or ice cubes (for thinning; optional)

1. Place all the ingredients in a blender and blend on high speed until smooth.
2. Thin with additional cold water or ice cubes, if desired.

MEXICAN CHOCOLATE SMOOTHIE

Ⓖ

Serves 1

8 ounces unsweetened coconut milk
¼ cup raw cacao powder
½ teaspoon alcohol-free pure vanilla extract
1 teaspoon ground cinnamon
¼ teaspoon freshly grated nutmeg
Pinch of cayenne pepper
½ cup frozen blueberries
1 tablespoon MCT oil (optional)

1. Place all the ingredients in a blender and blend on high speed until smooth.

Breakfast

GRAIN-FREE BREAKFAST CEREAL

Serves 1

1 tablespoon coconut oil
½ cup walnuts (preferably soaked overnight)
½ apple, seeded and diced
¼ cup shredded unsweetened coconut
¾ cup unsweetened coconut milk
½ teaspoon ground cinnamon
Pinch of organic stevia, for sweetening (optional)

1. Combine all the ingredients in a small saucepan and cook over medium-low heat for about 15 minutes.

OATMEAL POWER BOWL

Serves 1

1 cup steel-cut, certified gluten-free oats
1 small handful of blueberries
1 small handful of mixed nuts (almonds and walnuts)
1 teaspoon ground cinnamon
About ½ cup unsweetened coconut milk, or to taste

1. Cook the oats according to the package directions and add the remaining ingredients.

Dressings

BASIC SALAD DRESSING

Makes 4 servings

½ cup extra-virgin olive oil
2 tablespoons vinegar (cider, red wine, or balsamic)
½ teaspoon sea salt
½ teaspoon freshly ground black pepper

1. Whisk all the ingredients together.

LEMON OLIVE OIL VINAIGRETTE

Makes 4 servings

3 tablespoons freshly squeezed lime or lemon juice
¾ cup extra-virgin olive oil
Pinch each of sea salt and freshly ground black pepper

1. Whisk all the ingredients together.

CREAMY LEMON OLIVE OIL VINAIGRETTE

G

Makes 4 servings

3 tablespoons freshly squeezed lime or lemon juice
½ teaspoon Dijon mustard (optional)
¾ cup extra-virgin olive oil
Pinch each of sea salt and freshly ground black pepper

1. Whisk all the ingredients together.

ARTICHOKE OLIVE TAPENADE

G

Makes 8 servings

20 black olives, pitted
20 green olives, pitted
7 canned artichoke hearts
1 anchovy
1 garlic clove, minced
3 tablespoons shredded fresh basil
2 tablespoons extra-virgin olive oil
2 tablespoons freshly squeezed lemon juice

1. Place all the ingredients in a food processor and blend until combined. Serve on Flax Crackers (page 264).

CHIMICHURRI

G K

Makes 1 cup chimichurri

½ cup packed flat-leaf parsley
½ cup packed fresh cilantro
3 or 4 garlic cloves
2 tablespoons fresh oregano
2 tablespoons cider vinegar
Juice of ½ lemon
¾ cup extra-virgin olive oil
Pinch of red pepper flakes (optional)
1 teaspoon sea salt
¼ teaspoon freshly ground black pepper

1. Combine the parsley, cilantro, garlic, oregano, vinegar, lemon juice, olive oil, pepper flakes (if using), salt, and pepper and blend in a food processor or blender on high speed until just blended but not perfectly smooth.

Chimichurri goes great over any baked or grilled meat, such as steak, salmon, chicken, and pork. It has the perfect blend of fats from olive oils and the antioxidant effects from the herbs and spices.

Bread/Crackers

FLAX CRACKERS

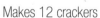

Makes 12 crackers

2 cups flax meal (ground flaxseeds)
½ teaspoon sea salt
1 teaspoon ground turmeric
Pinch of freshly ground black pepper

1. Preheat the oven to 400°F.
2. Mix all the ingredients together with ¾ cup of water in a food processor, adding a little extra water if necessary to achieve a doughlike consistency.
3. Spread out on parchment paper–lined baking sheet until the dough is ¼ inch thick or less. Carefully score the crackers (mark with the tip of a knife where the crackers will evenly break off after baking and cooling, not cutting all the way through).
4. Bake for 20 to 30 minutes, or until crisp and golden. When cool, break along the scores into individual crackers.

Flax seeds are rich in ALA omega-3 fatty acids, which, along with the turmeric in this recipe, provide a nice anti-inflammatory punch. It's preferable to grind flaxseeds at home rather than buying them already ground.

BUCKWHEAT BREAD

G

Makes 1 loaf

1¼ cups buckwheat flour
1 cup flax meal (ground flaxseeds)
½ teaspoon baking soda
½ teaspoon sea salt
¼ cup ground chia seeds
1½ cups warm water
2 tablespoons extra-virgin olive oil
1 tablespoon honey
1 tablespoon cider vinegar
Olive oil or coconut oil, for pan

1. Preheat the oven to 350°F.
2. Combine the buckwheat flour, flax meal, baking soda, and salt in a bowl, mixing with a whisk or fork.
3. Separately, combine the ground chia seeds and warm water in a blender and allow to sit for a minute. Then blend the olive oil, honey, and vinegar with the chia mixture.
4. Pour the wet ingredients into the dry ingredients, and stir until combined.
5. Oil a bread pan or baking dish with olive oil or coconut oil and then pour in the batter.
6. Bake for 30 to 40 minutes, or until a skewer inserted in the center comes out clean.

Lunch

DR. JOE'S FAVORITE SALAD

Serves 2

3 cups 50/50 mixed greens (50% spinach/50% mixed lettuce)
¼ cup blueberries or other berry, such as strawberries
½ cup chopped walnuts or almonds
½ ripe avocado, cubed
¼ cup Lemon Olive Oil Vinaigrette (page 261)

1. Combine all the ingredients in a large bowl and toss.
2. Add protein if serving as a main dish!

CONNECTICUT KALE SALAD

Serves 2

3 cups chopped kale
¼ cup toasted pine nuts or walnuts
¼ cup mixed strawberries and blueberries
¼ cup diced cucumber
¼ cup diced carrot
¼ cup Lemon Olive Oil Vinaigrette (page 261)

1. Combine all the ingredients in a large bowl and toss.

GREEN SALAD WITH POMEGRANATE SEEDS AND TOASTED WALNUTS

Serves 2

3 cups mixed greens
½ cup pomegranate seeds
½ cup crumbled walnuts
1 ripe avocado, cubed
¼ cup Creamy Lemon Olive Oil Vinaigrette (page 261)

1. Combine all the ingredients in a large bowl and toss.

ROASTED BEET AND ORANGE SALAD

Serves 4

12 small beets, peeled and cubed
½ cup extra-virgin olive oil, divided
3 oranges, peeled and cut into bite-size pieces
   (catch and reserve the juice)
4 cups chopped arugula
2 cups shredded radicchio
4 garlic cloves, minced
Sea salt and freshly ground black pepper
Extra-virgin olive oil (optional)

1. Preheat the oven to 350°F.
2. Toss the cubed beets with ¼ cup of the olive oil, and roast on a baking sheet for 20 to 25 minutes, or until tender.
3. In a large bowl, combine the beets, oranges, arugula, and radicchio.
4. In a smaller bowl, combine the remaining ¼ cup of olive oil and the reserved orange juice, minced garlic, and salt and pepper to taste. Drizzle over the salad and toss until combined. Add extra olive oil, if desired.

50/50 MIXED GREEN SALAD
WITH GRILLED SALMON

Ⓖ

Serves 2

2 cups 50/50 mixed greens (50% spinach/50% mixed lettuce)

1 cup sliced cucumber

½ cup cherry tomatoes

½ cup diced celery

½ cup sliced red onion

¼ cup almonds or sunflower seeds

¼ cup Lemon Olive Oil Vinaigrette Dressing (page 262)

1 (4-ounce) piece grilled salmon

1. Combine the greens, cucumber, tomatoes, celery, onion, and almonds in a large bowl and toss with the Lemon Olive Oil Vinaigrette Dressing.
2. Serve the grilled salmon atop the salad.

Vegetable Side Dishes

BAKED ACORN SQUASH

Serves 2

1 acorn squash
2 tablespoons ghee
Ground cinnamon
Freshly grated nutmeg
Sea salt and freshly ground black pepper

1. Preheat the oven to 400°F.
2. Cut the acorn squash in half and scoop out the seeds. Coat inside of each half with ghee (much of it will remain unmelted now but will, of course, melt in the oven), then (working with each half cut side up) sprinkle with cinnamon, nutmeg, salt, and pepper to taste.
3. Place the two halves, cut side up, in a baking dish. Bake for 45 to 60 minutes, or until tender when pierced with a fork.

LENTIL VEGGIE SAUTÉ

Serves 2 to 4

3 tablespoons ghee
1 cup dried lentils, soaked overnight
1 large zucchini, diced
2 carrots, diced
1 turnip, diced

1 onion, diced

4 garlic cloves, minced

4 Roma tomatoes

1 bunch spinach

¼ cup minced fresh cilantro

Sea salt and freshly ground black pepper

1. Heat the ghee in a large sauté pan over medium heat, then cook the lentils for 3 minutes.
2. Add the zucchini, carrots, turnip, onion, and garlic, plus about ¼ cup of water. Cook over low heat, covered, for 30 to 40 minutes, or until the lentils are tender.
3. Add the tomatoes and spinach and cook for an additional 3 minutes or until the spinach is wilted.
4. Remove from the heat, and add the cilantro plus salt and pepper to taste.

EGGPLANT MEDLEY

G

Serves 4

1 (1-pound) eggplant, cubed (about 5½ cups)

Sea salt

¼ cup extra-virgin olive oil

2 cups diced red onion

1 cup seeded and diced yellow bell pepper

1 cup seeded and diced orange bell pepper

2 garlic cloves, minced

1 (14-ounce) can diced tomatoes

Freshly ground black pepper

¼ cup minced fresh basll

1. Sprinkle the eggplant cubes with sea salt. Allow to sit for 5 minutes.

2. Heat the olive oil in a sauté pan over medium-low heat. Add the eggplant, onion, and bell peppers. Sauté for about 10 minutes, or until softened.
3. Add the garlic and tomatoes (including juice), and simmer for another 5 to 10 minutes.
4. Remove from the heat, add ground pepper to taste, and fold in the minced basil.

ROASTED VEGETABLES

Makes 2 servings

3 cups of three or more different vegetables (broccoli, cauliflower, brussels sprouts, asparagus, bell peppers, or eggplant)
¼ cup coconut oil

1. Preheat the oven to 400°F.
2. Chop all the vegetables into 1-inch pieces.
3. Combine all the ingredients in a bowl and then spread out on a baking sheet or roasting pan.
4. Roast for about 30 minutes, or until done.

Main Dishes

QUINOA PASTA WITH MEATBALLS

G

Serves 4

2 (8-ounce) boxes quinoa pasta
1 pound grass-fed ground beef
1 shallot, minced
¼ cup arugula, finely chopped
2 garlic cloves, minced
½ cup fresh herbs (such as oregano, basil, parsley, and/or sage), minced
1½ teaspoons sea salt
¼ cup extra-virgin olive oil
2 (14-ounce) cans diced tomatoes

1. Boil and drain the pasta according to the package directions.
2. Mix the ground beef in a bowl with the shallot, arugula, garlic, herbs, and salt. Roll into small balls.
3. Heat the olive oil in a sauté pan over medium heat. Brown the meatballs, turning every few minutes, then add the canned tomatoes (with juice). Continue to cook, covered, for about 8 minutes or until the meatballs are cooked through. Serve the meatballs and sauce on top of the pasta.

CHICKEN BREAST WITH PERSIMMON SALSA

Ⓖ

Serves 2 to 3

1 pound boneless, skinless chicken breast, cut into strips
¼ cup olive oil
¼ cup freshly squeezed lemon juice
Sea salt and freshly ground black pepper
3 ripe persimmons or mango, cut into small cubes
¼ to ½ jicama, cubed
2 tablespoons minced fresh cilantro
Juice of 1 lime
½ teaspoon cayenne pepper

1. Marinate the chicken breast in the olive oil, lemon juice, and salt and pepper for 30 minutes to several hours.
2. Grill or sauté over medium heat until cooked through, about 5 minutes.
3. In a bowl, combine the cubed persimmon, jicama, cilantro, lime juice, and cayenne. Serve on top of the grilled chicken.

COLORFUL QUINOA AND BLACK BEAN CASSEROLE

Ⓖ

Serves 3 to 4

2 tablespoons extra-virgin olive oil
2 cups cooked quinoa
1 (16-ounce) can black beans, drained and rinsed
2 cups seeded and diced orange and yellow bell pepper
1 teaspoon ground cumin
Sea salt and freshly ground black pepper
2 ripe avocados
1 cup shredded romaine lettuce
1 cup chopped tomato

1. Heat the olive oil over medium heat. Add the cooked quinoa, black beans, bell pepper, and cumin. Cook until the bell pepper is softened but still has some crispness.
2. Remove from the heat and pour into a serving bowl. Stir in salt and ground pepper to taste and the avocado, lettuce, and tomato until just combined. Serve immediately (or wait to add the avocado, lettuce, and tomato until just before serving).

TURKEY PATTIES

Ⓖ

Serves 4

1 pound ground turkey breast
¼ cup finely diced fennel
2 garlic cloves, minced
2 tablespoons finely minced fresh sage
1 teaspoon finely minced fresh thyme
1 teaspoon sea salt
½ teaspoon freshly ground black pepper
3 tablespoons extra-virgin olive oil, divided

1. In a large bowl, mix together the turkey, fennel, garlic, sage, thyme, salt, pepper, and 1 tablespoon of the olive oil. Shape into four or five patties.
2. Heat the remaining 2 tablespoons of olive oil over medium heat and cook the patties for about 4 minutes per side until browned and fully cooked through.

SPAGHETTI SQUASH PASTA WITH MEAT SAUCE

G

Serves 4

1 spaghetti squash, halved and seeded
2 tablespoons olive oil, plus more for brushing squash
1 onion, chopped
2 garlic cloves, crushed
1 pound lean beef
1 (28-ounce) can chopped tomatoes
1 teaspoon dried oregano
5 large basil leaves, chopped

1. Preheat the oven to 375°F.
2. Brush the inside of each half of the squash with olive oil. Place, cut side down, on a rimmed baking sheet.
3. Bake for about 40 minutes, or until you can easily pierce the squash with a fork. Let it cool for about 15 minutes. Then, using a fork, pull along the squash creating long "spaghetti" strands.
4. To make the sauce, place 2 tablespoons of olive oil in a large saucepan over medium-low heat. Add the chopped onion and crushed garlic and sauté until almost translucent and soft. Add the ground beef and sauté until browned.
5. Add the chopped tomatoes, oregano, and basil. Bring to a boil and then simmer over medium-low heat for 30 minutes.
6. Serve the spaghetti pasta with meat sauce.

BAKED SALMON WITH CHIVES

Ⓖ

Serves 2

2 (6-ounce) wild-caught salmon fillets
1 tablespoon ghee
2 teaspoons chopped fresh chives
Sea salt and freshly ground black pepper

1. Preheat the oven to 350°F.
2. Cut one large square of parchment paper for each fillet, and place each fillet in the center. Top each fillet with 1½ teaspoons of ghee, 1 teaspoon of chopped chives, and salt and pepper. Carefully fold the parchment paper over each fillet, tucking the edges underneath, to create an enclosed "packet."
3. Place the packets on a baking sheet. Bake for 15 to 20 minutes (depending on thickness), or until the fish flakes easily. Watch carefully so it doesn't overcook.
4. Unwrap the fish from the parchment paper and enjoy.

ROSEMARY GARLIC LAMB CHOPS

Ⓖ

Serves 2

2 teaspoons fresh rosemary, minced
2 garlic cloves, minced
Sea salt and freshly ground black pepper
2 (4- to 6-ounce) lamb chops, bone-in
2 tablespoons ghee

1. Rub the minced rosemary, garlic, salt, and pepper on each lamb chop.
2. Heat the ghee over medium heat in a sauté pan. Add the lamb chops and cook, covered, for about 4 minutes per side.
3. Remove from the heat when the center is just slightly pink.

ROASTED CHICKEN AND VEGETABLES

Ⓖ

Serves 4 to 6

2 tablespoons ghee, melted

3 garlic cloves, minced

1 teaspoon ground turmeric

1 teaspoon sea salt

½ teaspoon freshly ground black pepper

1 (5-pound) organic chicken

1 large onion, chopped

1 cup chopped carrot

1 cup mushrooms

1 cup brussels sprouts, cut in half

2 tablespoons coconut oil, melted

1. Preheat the oven to 375°F.
2. In a small bowl, mix together the melted ghee, garlic, turmeric, salt, and ½ teaspoon of pepper.
3. Place the chicken on a roasting rack, in a roasting pan, and coat the entire chicken with the ghee mixture, finishing with the chicken breast side being up.
4. Separately, in a large bowl, combine the onion, carrots, mushrooms, and brussels sprouts with the melted coconut oil and salt and pepper to taste. Once the vegetables are well coated, arrange them around the chicken in the roasting pan.
5. Bake for 75 to 90 minutes (depending on the size of the chicken).

STEAK WITH CHIMICHURRI SAUCE

Serves 2

2 (4- to 6-ounce) organic steaks, such as skirt steak,
   rib eye, or New York steak
Sea salt and freshly ground black pepper
Chimichurri Sauce (page 263)

1. Season the steak with salt and pepper and grill until the meat is well cooked
   on the outside, about 3 minutes per side. Transfer to a carving board and
   let rest for 5 minutes. Thinly slice the steak across the grain.
2. Spoon chimichurri sauce over each steak.

SLOW COOKER BUFFALO BRISKET

Serves 6 to 8

1 teaspoon extra-virgin olive oil
1 (3-pound) buffalo brisket
1 small onion, chopped
2 teaspoons chopped garlic
1 teaspoon dried basil
1 teaspoon dried oregano
1 teaspoon dried thyme
Sea salt and freshly ground black pepper
2 cups chicken bone broth (page 281) or chicken stock

1. Lightly coat the inside of a slow cooker with the olive oil and place the brisket in the bottom of the cooker.
2. Sprinkle with the onion, garlic, basil, oregano, and thyme; season with salt
   and pepper. Add the bone broth and 1 cup of water.
3. Cook on LOW until the brisket is tender, 6 to 10 hours, basting the meat
   several times to moisten.

SLOW COOKER BEEF BRISKET

G

Serves 4 to 6

1 (2- to 3-pound) grass-fed beef brisket
Paprika
Sea salt and freshly ground black pepper
2 carrots
2 celery stalks
2 turnips
5 mushrooms
1 large onion
¼ head broccoli
¼ head cauliflower
6 or 7 garlic cloves
1 (13-ounce) can diced tomatoes
2 cups beef bone broth (page 281)

1. Liberally sprinkle the paprika, salt, and pepper over both sides of the beef brisket. Set aside.
2. Chop all the vegetables and place in a slow cooker. Add the garlic, chopped tomatoes, and bone broth.
3. Place the beef brisket, whole, on top of vegetables, fat side up.
4. Cook on LOW for 8 to 10 hours. When the cooking is complete, remove the brisket, place it on a cutting board, and cut the entire brisket into cubes. Then, stir the brisket cubes back into the vegetables, and serve.

Soups/Stews

KALE SAUSAGE BEAN SOUP

Ⓖ

Serves 4

1½ pounds beef or pork sausage links
2 medium-size onions, diced
4 garlic cloves, minced
3 tablespoons extra-virgin olive oil
1 (16-ounce) can white beans, drained and rinsed
1 (16-ounce) can black beans, drained and rinsed
1 quart chicken bone broth (page 281)
1 bunch kale, chopped
1 teaspoon fennel seeds
Sea salt and freshly ground black pepper

1. Brown the sausage, onions, and garlic in the olive oil over medium-low heat in a heavy pot.
2. Add the beans and bone broth. Bring to a boil, lower the heat, and simmer, covered, for 1 hour.
3. Add the kale, fennel seeds, and salt and pepper to taste and simmer for about 15 more minutes. Serve hot.

BONE BROTH

Ⓖ Ⓚ

Makes about 8 cups broth

2 medium-size carrots
2 medium-size celery stalks
1 onion
2 organic pastured chicken carcasses, or 4 grass-fed beef bones)
Enough filtered water to cover the bones when they are in the pot
2 tablespoons coarse sea salt
1 tablespoon dried oregano
1 tablespoon dried thyme
1 teaspoon cider vinegar

1. The easiest way to make nutrient-dense bone broth is to use a slow cooker. Simply wash and coarsely halve/chop the vegetables, then place them and the bones in a slow cooker.
2. Fill the slow cooker with filtered water, then add the salt, oregano, thyme, and vinegar. Cook on LOW for 24 to 36 hours. Allow to cool a bit, then pour through a strainer to remove the vegetables and bones (which should be discarded).
3. You can freeze 2- to 3-cup portions for future use.

Dessert

LEMON COCONUT CUSTARD

Serves 2

2 cups unsweetened coconut milk

1 (1-tablespoon) packet unflavored gelatin, or 1½ packets for a firmer
consistency

½ cup freshly squeezed lemon juice

1 teaspoon alcohol-free pure vanilla extract

¾ teaspoon stevia powder

1. Warm the coconut milk, then stir in the unflavored gelatin until fully
dissolved.
2. Stir in the remaining ingredients, and then refrigerate for several hours or
until fairly firm.

Gelatin (the purified protein from beef collagen) is an excellent
healing food for the gut and joints. Be sure to purchase a good source
from grass-fed cows, such as Great Lakes brand.

KETOGENIC HEALING RECIPES

Beverages and Shakes

VANILLA SHAKE

Serves 1

4 ounces full-fat coconut milk
½ to 1 scoop protein powder
¼ cup hemp seeds
¼ cup chia seeds
1 tablespoon grass-fed gelatin (collagen)
1 teaspoon alcohol-free pure vanilla extract
Cold water or ice cubes (for thinning; optional)

1. Place all the ingredients in a blender and blend on high speed until smooth.

BERRY SHAKE

Serves 1

4 ounces full-fat coconut milk
4 ounces cold water
1 scoop protein powder

1 to 2 teaspoons chia seeds
¼ cup frozen berries
½ cup frozen kale or other greens
1 teaspoon ground cinnamon
1 tablespoon MCT oil (optional)

1. Place all the ingredients in a blender and blend on high speed until smooth.

CHOCOLATE SHAKE

Serves 1

4 ounces full-fat coconut milk
4 ounces cold water
¼ ripe avocado
¼ cup raw cacao powder
¼ cup frozen berries
1 teaspoon ground cinnamon
1 tablespoon MCT oil (optional)
A few ice cubes

1. Place all the ingredients in a blender and blend on high speed until smooth.

You can also add ½ cup of frozen greens instead of ice cubes.

CHOCOLATE COCONUT SHAKE

K

Serves 1

4 ounces full-fat coconut milk
4 ounces cold water
1 scoop protein powder
1 teaspoon raw cacao nibs
1 teaspoon chia seeds
¼ ripe avocado
½ cup shredded unsweetened coconut
1 tablespoon MCT oil (optional)

1. Place all the ingredients in a blender and blend on high speed until smooth.

CACAO-MINT SHAKE

K

Serves 1

4 ounces full-fat coconut milk
4 ounces cold water
1 scoop protein powder
Small handful of mint leaves
¼ ripe avocado
½ cucumber
1 teaspoon raw cacao nibs
1 tablespoon MCT oil (optional)

1. Place all the ingredients in a blender and blend on high speed until smooth.

KETO MATCHA GREEN TEA LATTE

Serves 1

1 teaspoon matcha powder
4 ounces hot water (not boiling)
4 ounces full-fat coconut milk, warmed
1 tablespoon MCT oil

1. Whisk the matcha powder and half of the hot water in a mug.
2. Pour the matcha mixture plus all the remaining ingredients into a blender and blend on high speed for just a few seconds.

Matcha tea is ten times more potent than other green teas
in terms of its antioxidants.

COCONUT TURMERIC TEA WITH GINGER

Serves 1

4 ounces full-fat coconut milk
4 ounces cold water
1 teaspoon ground turmeric, or 2 teaspoons grated fresh turmeric
1 teaspoon ground cinnamon
2 teaspoons minced fresh ginger

1. Place all the ingredients in a small pot over medium heat.
2. Once hot (but not boiling), transfer the mixture to a blender and blend on high speed until smooth.

KETOGENIC COFFEE

K

Serves 1

4 ounces full-fat coconut milk
4 ounces coffee
1 tablespoon coconut oil or MCT oil

1. Place all the ingredients in a blender and blend on high speed until smooth.

Breakfast

EGGS WITH SAUSAGE AND GREENS

Serves 2

½ pound sausage
2 large eggs
4 handfuls of spinach, kale, or 50/50 salad mix
   (50% spinach/50% mixed lettuce)

1. Slice the sausage into bite-size pieces, and sauté in a large skillet over medium heat for about 5 minutes, or until nearly cooked through.
2. Add the eggs to the pan and scramble with a fork. Cook for 1 minute.
3. Add the spinach, gently folding all three ingredients together in the pan, until the spinach is wilted.

POACHED EGGS WITH GHEE AND CILANTRO

Serves 1

White vinegar, for poaching
2 large eggs
Sea salt and freshly ground black pepper
1 teaspoon ghee
Minced fresh cilantro

1. Heat a pot of water (large enough to fit the two eggs) until it is simmering but not boiling. Add a dash of white vinegar.

2. Crack each egg into a small cup or ramekin. Swirl the water with a spoon to create a "whirlpool" in the water.
3. Gently slide each egg into the simmering water, and allow to cook for 4½ minutes, until the white is cooked and the yolk is still soft.
4. Use a slotted spoon to remove the eggs from the water and place on a plate.
5. Top with salt and pepper to taste, the ghee, and a sprinkle of fresh cilantro. Enjoy with a side salad or grilled radicchio.

SWEET ITALIAN SAUSAGE WITH SPICY BROCCOLI RABE

Serves 3 to 4

1 head broccoli rabe
¼ cup coconut oil or olive oil
1 garlic clove, chopped
1 to 2 teaspoons red pepper flakes
1 pound sweet Italian sausage links

1. Wash the broccoli rabe and then cut it into 2- to 3-inch-long pieces.
2. Heat the oil in a large skillet and lightly sauté the garlic.
3. Add the broccoli rabe and red pepper flakes. Sauté for about 5 minutes, or until the broccoli rabe has softened and wilted. Remove from the pan and set aside on a plate.
4. Add the sausage to the skillet and cook, turning often, until browned and cooked thoroughly.
5. Cut the sausage into 1-inch pieces and toss with the broccoli rabe.

Dressings

KETO COCONUT OIL SALAD DRESSING

K

Makes about 1 cup dressing

3 tablespoons cider vinegar
1 teaspoon lemon zest
2 tablespoons freshly squeezed lemon juice
½ teaspoon salt
⅓ cup extra-virgin olive oil
⅓ cup coconut oil, heated just until liquid

1. Place the vinegar, lemon zest and juice, and salt in a medium bowl and whisk until well combined.
2. While whisking continuously, slowly pour in the olive oil, then the coconut oil, until well blended.
3. Pour the dressing into a sealable container. Serve immediately.

KETO MAYO

K

Makes 1 cup mayonnaise

1 large egg
¼ small, ripe avocado
¾ cup extra-virgin olive oil
¼ cup MCT oil or coconut oil

2 teaspoons freshly squeezed lemon or lime juice
Pinch each of salt and freshly ground black pepper

1. Combine and blend all the ingredients with an immersion blender until the mayo is at the desired consistency (you can always add fresh herbs to flavor your mayo, too).

Lunch

POPEYE SPINACH SALAD WITH LEMON–OLIVE OIL VINAIGRETTE

Serves 4

4 cups baby spinach leaves,
  washed
½ cup thinly sliced red onion
4 strips cooked and crumbled
  bacon

¼ cup walnuts
¼ cup olive oil
Zest of 1 lemon, or 2 tablespoons
  freshly squeezed lemon juice

1. Divide the spinach leaves equally among four salad plates.
2. Lay the sliced red onion over the spinach and then sprinkle with the nuts and bacon crumbles.
3. To make the lemon–olive oil vinaigrette, whisk together the olive oil with the lemon zest or juice. Drizzle on top of each plate.

BUTTER LETTUCE SALAD WITH CREAMY SESAME DRESSING

Serves 2

1 small head butter lettuce, washed
½ cucumber, peeled and sliced into
  half-moons
¼ cup tahini

2 tablespoons olive oil
Juice of 1 lemon
  (about 3 tablespoons)

1. Shred the butter lettuce into large pieces and place in a large bowl.
2. Add the sliced cucumber.
3. In a separate small bowl or measuring cup, whisk together the tahini, olive oil, and lemon juice. Pour over the salad and toss until combined.

~~~~~~

This salad pairs well with canned sardines for a quick, easy, and nutritious lunch.

~~~~~~

TURKEY AVOCADO WRAP

Serves 2

Keto Mayo (page 290)
2 coconut wraps
4 slices roast turkey breast

4 to 6 sprigs of arugula
1 ripe avocado

1. Spread a dollop of Keto Mayo on each coconut wrap.
2. Top with the turkey, arugula, and avocado, roll up, and enjoy.

GRASS-FED BEEF BURGER

Serves 2

½ pound ground grass-fed beef
1 teaspoon dried thyme or oregano
Sea salt and freshly ground black
    pepper

Keto Mayo (page 290)
Avocado, for serving
Sliced tomato, for serving
2 romaine lettuce leaves

1. In a bowl, mix together the beef, thyme, and salt and pepper. Form into two patties.
2. Grill to your liking.
3. Top with Keto Mayo, avocado, and sliced tomato and wrap each burger in a romaine lettuce leaf.

Vegetable Side Dishes

TURMERIC-DUSTED BROCCOLI AND CAULIFLOWER

Serves 3 to 4

½ pound cauliflower, cut into 1-inch florets
½ pound broccoli, cut into 1-inch florets
6 tablespoons organic coconut oil
2 teaspoons ground turmeric
Sea salt and freshly ground black pepper

1. Preheat the oven to 350°F.
2. In a baking dish, toss together all the ingredients, seasoning with salt and pepper to taste.
3. Roast for 20 minutes, or until the cauliflower and broccoli are lightly browned in spots.
4. Serve warm or at room temperature.

ROASTED CAULIFLOWER WITH
KALAMATA OLIVES AND PINE NUTS

Serves 3 to 4

1 pound cauliflower, cut into 1-inch florets
2 tablespoons organic coconut oil
Sea salt and freshly ground black pepper
2 tablespoons pine nuts
½ cup chopped pitted kalamata olives
1 tablespoon chopped flat-leaf parsley

1. Preheat the oven to 350°F.
2. In a baking dish, toss the cauliflower with the coconut oil and season with salt and pepper.
3. Roast for 20 minutes, or until the cauliflower is lightly browned in spots.
4. Add the pine nuts, olives, and parsley and toss and roast for about 10 minutes longer, until the pine nuts are lightly toasted.
5. Serve warm or at room temperature.

"CREAMED" KALE OR SPINACH

K

Serves 3 to 4

1 tablespoon coconut oil, coconut butter, or ghee
1 large bunch kale or spinach, washed and shredded (or 1 bag prewashed kale or spinach)
⅓ cup full-fat coconut milk
Sea salt and freshly ground black pepper

1. Heat a large skillet over medium heat. Add the coconut oil.
2. Sauté the greens until softened, stirring often (spinach will cook in about 5 minutes; kale will need more like 20 to 25 minutes).
3. Add the coconut milk. Cook until the coconut milk thickens a bit, about 5 more minutes.
4. Season to taste with salt and pepper.

BRUSSELS SPROUTS WITH PANCETTA

Serves 4 or more

1½ pounds brussels sprouts, stems removed, halved
4 tablespoons olive oil or coconut oil
½ pound pancetta (1 thick slice), diced

1. Preheat the oven to 400°F.
2. In a large bowl, drizzle the halved brussels sprouts with 2 tablespoons of the olive oil, tossing to coat. Pour them onto a baking sheet and roast for 40 minutes.
3. While they're roasting, sauté the diced pancetta in remaining oil in a large, nonstick pan, cooking until golden brown. Remove the roasted brussels sprouts from the oven and pour the sautéed pancetta (plus any drippings) directly atop the brussels sprouts, tossing to combine.

Alternatively, you can use nitrite-free bacon for this dish.

ASPARAGUS WRAPPED WITH PROSCIUTTO

K

Serves 3 to 4

1 pound asparagus
2 tablespoons olive oil
2 tablespoons freshly squeezed lemon juice
Sea salt and freshly ground black pepper
¼ pound prosciutto di Parma

1. Wash the asparagus and trim the ends.
2. In a small bowl, mix together the olive oil, lemon juice, and salt and pepper to taste. Brush the asparagus spears with the olive oil mixture.
3. Grill the asparagus over medium heat for about 7 minutes (until just tender when pierced with a fork). Remove from the heat.
4. Separately, slice the prosciutto into long strips. Wrap the prosciutto around each individual asparagus spear.

If you don't have a grill, you can sauté the asparagus in a little
olive oil with a splash of water, over medium heat, covered,
until the asparagus is tender, about 5 minutes.

BITTER GREENS WITH ALMOND SAUCE

Ⓚ

Serves 4 to 6

8 cups shredded, washed greens (such as a combination of dandelion, collard, chicory, and mustard greens)
2 tablespoons coconut oil
3 tablespoons almond butter
2 tablespoons full-fat coconut milk
2 tablespoons freshly squeezed lime juice
1 tablespoon coconut aminos
1 garlic clove, minced

1. Sauté the greens in the coconut oil over medium heat, covered, for about 8 minutes.
2. In a small bowl, whisk together the almond butter, coconut milk, lime juice, coconut aminos, and garlic.
3. When the greens are cooked, transfer to a serving bowl and mix the sauce into the greens.

Main Dishes

GREEN TEA POACHED SALMON WITH ESCAROLE

Ⓚ

Serves 2

2 cups boiling water
4 green tea bags
1 tablespoon grated fresh ginger
1 tablespoon coconut aminos
3 tablespoons coconut oil, divided
2 (8-ounce) wild-caught salmon fillets
1 head escarole, coarsely chopped

1. Steep the green tea in the hot water for about 4 minutes. Remove the tea bags, and stir the ginger and coconut aminos into the liquid.
2. In a skillet, heat 2 tablespoons of the coconut oil over medium-low heat, and sear both sides of the salmon for 2 to 3 minutes per side.
3. Place the salmon in the skillet, skin side down (if it still has the skin), and add the tea mixture. Bring to a boil, then lower the heat, cover, and poach for 7 to 8 minutes, or until salmon flakes easily.
4. In a separate sauté pan, heat the remaining 1 tablespoon of coconut oil over medium heat, add the chopped escarole plus 1 tablespoon of water, and cook for 4 to 5 minutes.
5. To serve, divide the escarole between two dinner plates, and use a slotted spoon to lift the salmon out of the poaching liquid and onto the bed of escarole.

MACADAMIA-CRUSTED COD

Serves 3 to 4

1 cup full-fat coconut milk
2 eggs
1½ cups coconut flour
½ teaspoon sea salt
1¼ cups coarsely ground
   macadamia nuts

1½ pounds cod fillet,
   cut into 2-inch strips
4 to 6 tablespoons
   coconut oil

1. In one bowl, whisk together the coconut milk and eggs.
2. Combine the coconut flour and salt in a second bowl.
3. Place the ground macadamia nuts in a third bowl.
4. Carefully dip each strip of cod into the coconut milk mixture, then in the coconut flour, then back to the coconut milk mixture, and then into the ground macadamia nuts.
5. Heat the coconut oil over medium heat, then sauté each cod strip for 3 to 5 minutes per side, until the crust is nicely browned and the fish flakes easily.

SHRIMP WITH COCONUT CREAM SAUCE AND ZUCCHINI NOODLES

Serves 2 to 3

1 (13-ounce) can full-fat coconut milk
3 tablespoons ghee
¼ cup arrowroot flour
½ cup walnuts, finely ground
Sea salt and freshly ground
   black pepper

1½ pounds spiralized
   zucchini "noodles"
1 pound shrimp, cooked

1. In a saucepan, combine the coconut milk, ghee, arrowroot, ground walnuts, and salt and pepper to taste and heat, whisking continuously, until thickened.
2. Once thickened, add the zucchini noodles plus the cooked shrimp, and simmer for about 3 minutes.

This coconut cream sauce can be used for any
cooked chicken, fish, and/or vegetables.

SLOW COOKER CHICKEN CURRY

Serves 4 to 6

2 tablespoons ghee
1 tablespoon finely chopped fresh
   ginger
2 garlic cloves, minced
1 (13-ounce) can full-fat coconut milk
½ cup water or chicken bone broth
   (page 281)
½ teaspoon ground turmeric
2 teaspoons ground coriander
1 teaspoon curry powder
Sea salt and freshly ground black
   pepper

3 medium-size zucchini,
   cut into half-moons
3 medium-size summer
   squash, cut into
   half-moons
2 pounds boneless chicken
   thighs
Minced fresh cilantro, for
   garnish

1. Heat the ghee in a sauté pan over medium heat and add the ginger and garlic. Cook, stirring continuously, for less than a minute.
2. Place the ghee mixture and all the other ingredients, except chicken and cilantro, in a slow cooker. Stir to mix the ingredients before adding chicken thighs last.
3. Cook on LOW for 7 to 9 hours.
4. Serve with freshly minced cilantro.

Soups/Stews

CHICKEN AVOCADO LIME SOUP

Serves 4

2 tablespoons olive oil

1 onion, diced

½ jalapeño pepper, seeded and minced (optional)

2 garlic cloves, minced

1½ to 2 quarts chicken bone broth (page 281) or chicken stock

½ teaspoon ground cumin

1 to 2 Roma tomatoes, seeded and diced

1½ pounds boneless skinless chicken breast

Sea salt and freshly ground black pepper (optional)

⅓ cup chopped fresh cilantro

3 medium-size, ripe avocados, peeled, seeded, and cubed

Juice of 2 limes

1. Heat the olive oil in a large pot over medium heat, and then add the diced onion and jalapeño (if using). Sauté for 2 to 5 minutes, or until the onion is tender and translucent.
2. Add the garlic and cook for another 30 seconds.
3. Next, add the bone broth, cumin, tomatoes, chicken breasts, and salt and pepper (if using). Bring to a boil over high heat, then lower the heat to a simmer. Cover with a lid while the chicken cooks. The cooking time depends on thickness of the breasts and may be 15 to 30 minutes. When done, it should be easy to shred the chicken with a fork.
4. Lower the heat to low, then remove the chicken breasts and allow them to cool for 5 to 10 minutes. When cool, shred the chicken with your fingers and return it to the pot. Add the cilantro.
5. Ladle into individual bowls, then top each with some of the avocado cubes (less than half of an avocado per serving) and a generous squeeze of lime juice.

SLOW COOKER LAMB STEW

Ⓚ

Serves 6 to 8

2 to 3 pounds lamb stew meat
¼ cup arrowroot flour
¼ cup bacon fat or tallow
1 onion, diced
3 celery stalks, chopped
2 carrots, chopped
1 cup diced rutabaga
1 cup diced turnip
1 (8-ounce) can diced tomatoes
1 teaspoon dried rosemary
1 teaspoon dried thyme
1 teaspoon ground cumin
1 teaspoon sea salt
¼ teaspoon freshly ground black pepper
3 cups beef bone broth (page 281)

1. Coat the lamb with the arrowroot, place in large, heavy-bottomed saucepan and brown in the bacon fat or tallow over medium heat. Once browned, remove from the heat.
2. Place all the vegetables and seasonings in a slow cooker. Top with the browned meat.
3. Using some of the bone broth, deglaze the pan you just used to brown the meat, and pour it off into the slow cooker, adding all the remaining bone broth as well.
4. Cook on LOW for 8 to 10 hours.

Dessert

ALMOND BUTTER TREATS

Makes about 12 treats

1 cup almond butter
½ cup coconut oil, melted
2 tablespoons ghee, melted
½ cup shredded unsweetened coconut
½ cup coconut flour
2 teaspoons ground cinnamon
1 teaspoon stevia powder

1. Place all the ingredients in a food processor and process until combined.
2. Roll into bite-size balls and place on a rimmed baking sheet in a single layer. Place in freezer for 1 to 2 hours.
3. Continue to store in the freezer until ready to eat.

AVOCADO CHOCOLATE MOUSSE

Serves 2

1 (5.4-ounce) can coconut cream
½ ripe avocado
¼ cup raw cacao powder
½ teaspoon ground cinnamon (optional)
Liquid stevia (can use flavored stevia, such as orange or mint)
Blackberries or pomegranate seeds, for garnish

1. Place the can of coconut cream in the fridge for about 8 hours. Without shaking the can, open it, and scoop out the thickened cream into a food processor or blender, discarding the remaining water.
2. Add the avocado, cacao powder, cinnamon, and stevia and blend.
3. Scoop into individual ramekins, and top with blackberries or pomegranate seeds.

MINT CHOCOLATE CHIP ICE CREAM

Serves 4

2 large, ripe avocados
1 (13-ounce) can full-fat coconut milk
3 drops mint-flavored liquid stevia
½ cup fresh mint leaves
¼ cup MCT oil
1 cup cacao nibs

1. Scoop the avocado flesh into a food processor.
2. Add all the other ingredients, except the cacao nibs, and blend until smooth.
3. Transfer to an ice-cream maker and process as instructed by the manufacturer. Then, add the cacao nibs. If you don't have an ice-cream maker, transfer to a bowl after blending in the food processor, then stir in cacao nibs and place in the freezer until well chilled.

APPENDIX B: HEALING PAIN NUTRIENT PROTOCOLS

For Everyone		
Supplement	**Dosage**	**Notes**
Multivitamin/mineral	2x/day	Twice daily multivitamin and mineral.
Omega-3 fatty acids EPA and DHA	3000–5,000 mg/day	Used to decrease inflammation, modulate pain, regulate blood sugar and cholesterol levels.
Vitamin D3	1000–2,000 IU daily	Deficiencies of less than 50 ng/mL have been associated with inflammation, leaky gut, decreased healing, autoimmunity, migraines and musculoskeletal pain.

Inflammation/Immune Support		
Supplement	**Dosage**	**Notes**
Curcumin	500 mg 2x/day	Contain natural plant-based antioxidant, anti-inflammatory, and immune stimulating properties to modulate proinflammatory pathways. Positive effects have been noted with decreased reactive oxygen species, NF-kB, leukotriene and prostaglandins, blood sugar and fatty acid rebalancing.
Resveratrol	500 mg 2x/day	
N-acetyl-D-glucosamine	500 mg daily	
Ginger	200 mg 2x/day	
Skullcap	100 mg daily	
Proteolitic enzymes	200 mg 2x/day	
Boswellia	200 mg 2x/day	
Andrographis paniculata	2,000 mg 2x/day	

4R Gut-Healing Program		
Supplement	Dosage	Notes
Remove Botanical for treating SIBO	1 capsule daily	Botanical blend including extracts from berbine (Berberis vulgaris), oregano (Origanum vulgare), grapefruit (Citrus paradisi).
Replace Digestive enzyme	1 capsule with meals	Enzyme blend including betaine HCl, amylase, protease, pepsin, lactase, and lipase.
Repopulate Probiotics	1–2 capsules daily	50–100 billion IU per capsule blend of live cultures containing lactobacillis and bifidobacterium strains. Avoid probiotics that are not gluten, soy, corn, and diary free.
Repair L-glutamine	1–2 g 2x/day	An essential amino acid needed by the body for repair of the digestive tract and enterocytes in the gut. L-L-glutamate, in addition to fiber, serves as a fuel precursor for colonocytes.
Gut formula	Once daily	Gut repair formulas include a mix of vitamins, minerals, and herbs including: deglycyrrhizinaed licorice, aloe vera extract, slippery elm, marshmallow, MSM, chamomile, mucin, okra extract, quercetin, zinc, n-acetyl glucosamine, vitamin D.

Joint Healing		
Supplement	Dosage	Notes
Glucosamine sulfate	1,000 mg daily	All are important nutrients and precursors for healthy joint tissue, structure, and function and found in cartilage, ligaments, tendons, and connective tissue.
Chondroitin sulfate	1,000 mg daily	
MSM (methulsulfonylmethane)	250 mg daily	
Collagen peptides	7 g daily	
Hyaluronic acid	40 mg daily	

Tension/Tightness		
Supplement	Dosage	Notes
Valerian root	200 mg 2x/day	Extracts of valerian and other plant-based extracts may help reduce muscle pain and muscle tension through inducing relaxation, reducing anxiety, and possibly mild sedation of the nervous system.
Passion flower	200 mg 2x/day	
Lemon balm	100 mg 2x/day	
Magnesium	500 mg 2x/day	

Stress and Sleep		
Supplement	Dosage	Notes
GABA	200 mg as needed	Gamma-aminobutyric acid is a naturally occurring neurotransmitter in the brain, providing calm and reducing mild stress and anxiety.
L-theanine	200 mg 1–2x/day	An amino acid found in green tea, reduces anxiety and relieves stress by inducing relaxation without drowsiness.
5-HTP	50 mg daily	A protein building block for the amino acid tryptophan and is a precursor for serotonin and melatonin. Should be taken along with vitamin B6. Helpful with relaxation as well as sleep.
Melatonin	0.3–3 mg, as needed	An important antioxidant scavenging free radicals and supporting a healthy immune and stress response. Melatonin can be taken before bed or in divided doses at dinner and then bedtime.

Muscle/Tissue Repair		
Supplement	**Dosage**	**Notes**
Branched-Chain amino acids (BCAAs) (Leucine, isoleucine, valine + L-glutamine)	5–10 g	Branched-chain amino acids along with L-glutamine stimulate muscle synthesis even in the absence of resistance training, making them essential in those who are unable to exercise but are at risk for muscle loss (sarcopenia). BCAAs are also essential in sports nutrition— enhancing muscle building and recovery in athletes. BCAAs can also prevent sarcopenia post-operatively, after a traumatic injury and muscle catabolism associated with inflammatory diseases.

SOURCES

ABOUT DR. JOE TATTA

Website: http://www.drjoetatta.com
    The Healing Pain Program: www.healingpainprogram.com
    Healing Pain Support Group: www.drjoetatta.com/group
    Healing Pain Podcast. http://www.drjoetatta.com/podcasts
    Healing Pain Summit: http://www.thehealingpainsummit.com
    Active Healing Store: http://www.store.drjoetatta.com

SOCIAL MEDIA

Facebook: https://www.facebook.com/JoeTattaPT/
    Twitter: @DrJoeTatta
    Linkedin: Dr Joe Tatta, DPT
    Speaking Engagements: support@drjoetatta.com

PRODUCTS FOR MINIMIZING STRESS AND PAIN

Sauna for Detoxification
    http://www.sunlighten.com
Heart Math
    http://www.heartmath.com
Muse: The Brain-Sensing Headband for Meditation
    http://www.choosemuse.com

FUNCTIONAL LAB TESTING

Direct Labs
    www.directlabs.com

Cyrex Labs
  www.cyrexlabs.com
Diagnostechs
  http://www.diagnostechs.com

DR. JOE'S FAVORITE BOOKS TO HEAL PAIN

Cracking the Metabolic Code. James B. LaValle, RPh, CCN, ND
Explain Pain. David Butler, PT, DEd
It Starts with Food. Dallas Hartwig and Melissa Hartwig
Less Pain, Fewer Pills. Beth Darnall, PhD
The Autoimmune Solution. Amy Myers, MD
Why Isn't My Brain Working? Datis Kharrazian, DHSc, DC, MS

ORGANIZATION AND SUPPORT GROUPS

The American Physical Therapy Association
  www.APTA.org
National Association of Nutrition Professionals
  www.NANP.org
Association for Contextual Behavioral Science
  https://contextualscience.org
American Association of Drugless Practitioners
  http://aadp.net
American Academy of Pain Medicine
  http://www.painmed.org
American Chronic Pain Association
  https://theacpa.org

NUTRITION RESOURCES

Thrive Market
  Organic products at wholesale prices
  https://thrivemarket.com
Vital Choice Wild Seafood and Organics
  www.VitalChoice.com
National Farmers Market Directory
  https://www.ams.usda.gov
The Environmental Working Group
  https://www.ewg.org

ACKNOWLEDGMENTS

Writing a book requires the collaboration from many great minds, and I have had the support of many throughout this process. I would like to express my appreciation to all the talented people who contributed to the creation of this work. First, to my agent Coleen O'Shea, who recognized the importance of the book and message. Coleen, our timing was perfect and in many ways ahead of the curve. To Lara Asher, for helping me mold and create this work as if it were her own. Your patience, guidance, and support were invaluable. Thank you for helping hone my message. To my editor Dan Ambrosio, Claire Ivett, and the entire team at Da Capo Press. It was great working with you all. Your expertise made the literary process "painless" and smooth. A special thank you to Bill Westmoreland for the photography and video design.

It took me forty years to find amazing mentors without whom this book would not have been possible. To Brendon Burchard, who taught me to think bigger and reactivated that human drive that makes one feel alive. This book was conceived though your mentorship and inspiration. To JJ Virgin, for being an incredible role model and for encouraging me to act boldly. You are a true leader in the health space. To all my friends in the mindshare community, especially Dr. Nicole Beurkens, Dr. Susan Albers, Dr. Joan Rosenberg, Dr. Susanne Bennett, Dr. Anne Shippy, Dr. Nalini Chilkov, Dr. Robin Benson, Dr. Sara Gottfried, Dr. Alan Christianson, and Dr. Kellyann Pertucci. Each of you is a visionary and inspires me to do greater work. I am blessed to be on this journey with you. A special thank-you to Dr. David Asomaning. Dave, you have been my inner genius when I needed it the most and I am forever grateful for your guidance.

To the greatest parents anyone could ask for. Dad, your affection and humor has always filled my life. You are my toughest patient but one worth fighting for. Keep up the good work! To my mom, an incredible nurse who dedicated her life to healing others and inspired me to pursue a career in which I would do the same. The world needs more great nurses like you! Both of you taught me to dream big and build a solid foundation under those dreams. This book is yet another brick in that foundation.

A special thank you to the thousands of professionals and patients I have had the honor to work with over the past twenty years. Thank you for allowing me to care for and mentor you to greater health and success. Together we can end our pain epidemic.

Finally, my husband, Jeorge, has always believed in and supported my work. You valiantly stand by my side and support me through life's challenges and triumphs. Thank you for enduring my frequent travel and hours spent with my head lost in the computer researching and writing. You graciously endured my madness throughout this process and tolerated the piles of paper scattered around our home. I promise to clean up the paper soon, just in time to begin the next book!

INDEX

ABOUT THE AUTHOR

Dr. Joe Tatta is a doctor of physical therapy, board-certified nutrition specialist, and functional medicine practitioner who specializes in treating persistent pain and lifestyle-related musculoskeletal, metabolic, and autoimmune health issues. His mission is to create a new paradigm around treating persistent pain and reverse our global pain epidemic. He is the creator of the Healing Pain Online Summit and The Healing Pain Podcast designed to broaden the conversation around natural strategies toward solving persistent pain. He is currently in private practice in New York City and also provides Online Health Consulting to help people achieve their optimal level of vitality and freedom from chronic disease. Learn more by visiting www.drjoetatta.com and www.healingpainprogram.com.